The Fibromyalgia Cure

"Dr. Dryland changed my mind about fibromyalgia. I was one of those people who believed that it was a cop-out diagnosis, that it was a catchall – now I don't. Now I understand it. Dr. Dryland has researched it, he has legitimized it, and he's changing the minds of other professionals."

– Jude S., Registered Nurse and Patient

"Dr. Dryland gave me back my life. I feel great!"

– Pat C., Patient

"I haven't felt like this for several years. I think he's a fabulous doctor!"

– Mildred S., Patient

"I find Dr. Dryland to be a doctor with incredible integrity and a genuine concern for his patients. He helped to change my life – completely turn it around!"

– Ali D., Patient

"I had no hope, but now I do have hope! My experience is that it worked. It's working because I am getting help. I am feeling better!"

– Marta S., Patient

"Dr. Dryland saved my life!"

– Vicky G., Patient

THE FIBROMYALGIA CURE

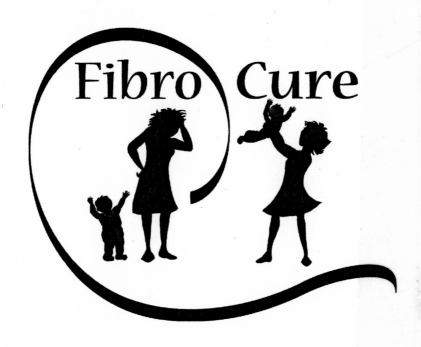

Fibro Cure

David Dryland, M.D.

This book is dedicated to:

Amelia and Alexander, my children –
They are my love and my life

All of my patients –
by sharing your suffering you revealed to me
what fibromyalgia truly is

Jerry Garcia –
for setting me free

FOREWORD
by Dr. Andrew J. Holman, M.D.

No one ever sets out to be a fibromyalgia specialist.

Those of us in healthcare choose to participate in patient care for a variety of reasons, but not everyone has the stamina and desire to tackle our most daunting medical disorders. One can make significant contributions, to science, to the health and well being of our patients and to career fulfillment, but still not engage in the daily stress of trying to cure the untreatable. Historically, treating fibromyalgia has not been for everyone.

But, on occasion, there are physicians and other caregivers who rise above their peers to fight the losing battle and support the less popular and forgotten. Many physicians still hope that fibromyalgia will simply go away, so that they can get back to real medicine. Others remain skeptical of its very existence despite the 10 million Americans afflicted. A smaller group, for individual reasons of their own, choose the road less traveled, a road that may someday lead to a cure for fibromyalgia.

David Dryland, M.D., has chosen such a path and has demonstrated his conviction to this cause by sharing his views with you in *The Fibromyalgia Cure.*

I first met David at an informal Sunday morning breakfast at a medical meeting in 2001. While discussing very new research relating to the use of dopamine agonists for the treatment of fibromyalgia, I mentioned that my life was "getting easier." This sentiment seems to have resonated with David. New medications to address an overactive stress, or the 'fight-or-flight' response, were improving sleep quality and decreasing pain for patients with fibromyalgia. Life in the office had been a misery, since very little I had to offer these patients provided much benefit. While my patients with rheumatoid arthritis were doing well, I would see 10-12 patients with fibromyalgia every day, and nothing worked. Side effects were pervasive and during every stressful holiday or Pacific storm, my staff and I would be overwhelmed by phone calls from desperate patients in flare.

As this stress response began to be understood and addressed biochemically, fibromyalgia pain and fatigue waned. Finally, a few patients recovered completely. That was when we got to work to find out what had changed. Their stress response had changed. Their hair trigger for an excessive stress and arousal response had dissipated and patients finally slept normally. Previously, patients might improve, but were rarely completely symptom free. It was the first complete responders that revealed the essence of fibromyalgia.

At about the same time, animal stress models and basic science research on the central neurotransmitter, dopamine was emerging. The confluence of these events set in motion the new approach to fibromyalgia revolving around dopamine and its role as a regulator of basic human housekeeping functions, including sleep, temperature regulation, bowel motility, stomach acid production, heart rate, blood pressure and the most basic stress fight-or-flight responses. In those first complete responders, all of these body functions improved simultaneously as their fibromyalgia pain and fatigue resolved.

Over a century ago, endocrinology was born when physicians learned about how hormones control so many human functions. The ability of the body to regulate itself was a new and exciting concept. The thyroid, adrenal glands, pituitary and other endocrine glands became a central area of research for illnesses that seems almost trivial in the 21st century. Today, we simply check blood tests to diagnose what were impossibly complex disorders years ago. Research on dopamine and how the brain regulates human function will become similarly pivotal. In fact, through the pituitary and hypothalamus, the endocrine system coordinates its control of human homeostasis with the same system that controls fight-or-flight: the autonomic nervous system. These two systems are remarkably interconnected.

Consequently, it should not be surprising that we learn so much more about ourselves when we explore how dopamine regulates this counterpart to the endocrine system. Both systems work in concert to keep us well and to deal with assaults to our health, such as infection, cancer, injury or other stressors. General interest in brain neurotransmitters may have been popularized by serotonin, but dopamine may turn out to be so much more important. It will take some time for these new concepts to be digested by the medical world at large, but this is a very exciting time historically and remarkably significant for those with fibromyalgia.

Finally, I would emphasize that, while important, an encyclopedic memory is not the highest quality of a physician or any profession that deals with challenges. I teach the residents and medical students that their primary resource is courage. Courage provides the strength to persevere, to empathize and to care for patients, even when we all fear failure. Courage supports honesty when the caregiver has to tell the patient that they have no answers. It also takes courage to consider new ideas.

While patients clearly suffer more than their physicians, relentless failure can bury one's altruism. Under such circumstances, physicians loose faith in themselves and their ability. And, physicians abhor failure. Perhaps, this is partly why many run from fibromyalgia or are too eager to challenge its existence. Thankfully, Dr. Dryland can be counted among those who embraced adversity and continued to search for answers to this epic challenge.

Andrew J. Holman, M.D.
Assistant Clinical Professor of Medicine
University of Washington
Pacific Rheumatology Associates

March 11, 2005

CONTENTS

Foreword by Andrew J. Holman, M.D.   vi

Introduction   xi

Chapter 1 Three Steps to Diagnosing Fibromyalgia 1

Chapter 2 What is Fibromyalgia? 7
Why Does it Hurt?

Chapter 3 Unveiling the Causes of Fibromyalgia 27

Chapter 4 What Will Fibromyalgia Do to Me? 47

Chapter 5 What Can I Do About Fibromyalgia? 71

Chapter 6 Explaining Fibromyalgia 99

Chapter 7 Moving Beyond Fibromyalgia: 111
Your Plan for a Cure

Appendix for Healthcare Providers   133

Notes, Bibliography   148

~

INTRODUCTION

The key to fibromyalgia lies within these pages. You will not simply find the next thing to try, the next gimmick or the next disappointment. Within this book is a revolutionary, yet scientifically correct, explanation of exactly what fibromyalgia is, why it hurts, and what you can do about it both naturally and with the help of medications.

You'll use my easy to follow guidelines to see if you have fibromyalgia. This self-diagnosis tool is the first of its kind. Next, you'll get an easy-to-understand, clear explanation of what fibromyalgia is and why you suffer. Later in the book you'll get to pick from four treatment approaches designed to help you reduce or completely alleviate your symptoms.

By the time you have finished this book, you'll have the tools you need to understand how you can eliminate the symptoms of fibromyalgia and, as my patients tell me, "get your life back!"

If this all sounds just a little too good to be true, let me give you some background on how I arrived at this point. While training as a rheumatologist at Yale University I learned that rheumatologists, in addition to treating the auto-immune diseases, are generally supposed to determine why people hurt and provide treatment. But upon entering clinical practice, I found that even though millions of people suffer from fibromyalgia, very little was known about the nature of the disease or how to treat it.

I didn't learn a lot about fibromyalgia in medical school, but my professors helped instill a lifelong passion for science. This love of science has served me well. I've used a broad spectrum of scientific data to help develop practical fibromyalgia treatments. But even more importantly is the one-on-one time I've spent with a large number of fibromyalgia patients. They have taught me much about fibromyalgia – probably at least as much as all of the current existing research.

Through their stories, I came to realize that fibromyalgia is not a disease, but a response our bodies have developed to protect us in times of danger. I came to understand that fibromyalgia patients are stuck in a vicious cycle of elevated adrenaline due to our ancient "fight or flight response."

Over the years I began to categorize the conditions that have caused people to get stuck in the cycle and ultimately help patients identify their own successful treatment plans. I began to counsel patients and found that when provided with insights into what was actually happening to them and why - the majority were able to heal themselves. I also provided medication as necessary to ease symptoms while people progressed through their personalized treatment plan. Compared with many current approaches to fibromyalgia treatment, the success rates are incredible!

I think this is partially because I can identify with my patients and their struggles since I too once had to cure my own fibromyalgia. When I graduated from Yale, I had trouble deciding what type of medical practice I wanted. I wasn't happy in my first job. I moved a few times, and had to relocate my young family. I had just purchased a house. It was a stressful time for us as our dreams crumbled and I found myself having to start all over again.

It was at this point that I began to show signs of extreme stress. My wife and I argued. My legs grew restless at night. I also suffered bouts of uncontrollable itching. It was humiliating, especially since nobody, including the physicians I worked with, could help me.

If you have fibromyalgia, you know exactly what I am talking about. You have these strange things happening to your body and you want answers. You want to DO something. All of my medical tests came back normal. Still, I was losing sleep and itching for hours at night. At the time, I never dreamed I had fibromyalgia, but later I discovered I did and eventually figured out how to cure my symptoms.

My own breakthrough came when I began to take fibromyalgia patients more seriously. I questioned them about everything in their lives. I learned from them. I made lists of what was wrong with them and what might have caused their problems. Things began to make sense and I finally began to understand what was really happening and why.

The lessons I learned, both as a sufferer of fibromyalgia and as a rheumatologist responsible for the care of fibromyalgia patients, gave me the keys to start effectively counseling patients. More often than not, my patients benefited as a result.

As I became known locally as a physician willing to treat fibromyalgia, I began to receive referrals for more severe cases. These were people who were miserable and were stuck in a vicious cycle where pain caused more stress, more depression and the loss of sleep – leading inevitably to even more intense fibromyalgia symptoms. In many cases, these patients were unable to work on the root causes of their fibromyalgia even when provided with an appropriate plan and the best available medications.

I soon realized it was not particularly useful to tell someone who was suffering, crying and barely able to get out of bed that they should try to "be less stressed and get good sleep." I realized that a common denominator with all of my patients was increased adrenaline, the chief chemicals of the fight or flight response. I somehow needed to get their adrenaline to cycle normally.

That's when I met Dr. Andrew Holman. We were among only a few clinical rheumatologists studying fibromyalgia. Dr. Holman was more focused on the severe cases and had been astute enough to apply high doses of restless legs medications in these instances. Restless legs syndrome is frequently seen in patients with fibromyalgia and is tied to an altered dopamine metabolism and increased adrenaline levels. The medications used to treat the restless legs syndrome are called dopamine agonists: basically adrenaline in a bottle. When a person suffering from fibromyalgia takes high doses of these at night, their adrenaline level can be regulated allowing the body to start perceiving sensations in a normal way again. When this happens, the "fight or flight response" subsides, relinquishing control of your life. This medical regimen has proved a great help for a large number of my patients who have tried it. The complete protocol is discussed in detail in the provider appendix.

The best way to cure fibromyalgia is to first understand what you have, identify your particular causes and then start to work on them so that your fight or flight response is no longer activated.

When you have finished this book you will understand:

1) **Your particular causes and how they trigger your fibromyalgia.**
2) **Which symptoms you can attribute to fibromyalgia, and which you cannot.**
3) **What to tell your family, friends, and co-workers.**
4) **How to treat your own fibromyalgia or provide your healthcare professional with tools that can assist your treatment.**

The American College of Rheumatology (ACR) has been particularly aggressive in insisting that rheumatologists refuse to see patients with fibromyalgia. In part, this is because there is a national shortage of rheumatologists, and within our current legal climate, this situation is likely to worsen. At the same time, our population is aging and growing.

This means that patients suffering from some of the most serious cases of arthritis, such as rheumatoid arthritis, have had to wait as long as several months to see a rheumatologist. The ACR, as a consequence, feels rheumatologists should reserve their time primarily for those patients with crippling diseases — consulting with people with less physically destructive problems only as time permits. This seems reasonable enough. However, with the worsening national shortage of medical specialists, this also doesn't leave much room for people suffering from fibromyalgia.

The implications of this situation may prove profound for the individuals who suffer with fibromyalgia, for the professionals who treat it, as well as for those responsible for setting health care policies. That's because a growing number of untreated cases of fibromyalgia will likely result not only in more suffering, but also in more disabilities and insurance claims. My hope in writing this book is that people will be empowered to help themselves as much as possible regardless of how the health care community decides to respond.

David Dryland, M.D.

CASE STUDY

FRED L.

Sixty-nine year old Fred L. had been suffering with pain most of his life when finally he discovered Dr. Dryland. Here's what he says about his experience.

MAJOR SYMPTOMS

"The main one was pain – it moved throughout my body. It came and went, sometimes very severe. It was mostly in my hips or back, or my left shoulder. I have seen other doctors; they all looked at me like I was crazy when I talked to them about having been in pain all my life. I've had it my whole life!"

RESULTS

"When I went to Dr. Dryland, first and foremost, he didn't look at me like I was crazy. I thought, finally, I've got somebody who had some idea about what I'm going through in life. He had done his research; he knew what I was talking about. I fit in the category to say that I had fibromyalgia. I used to be tense, sometimes very irritable if the pain got really bad. Now I don't have that kind of pain anymore. It began to change the way in which I present myself."

~

CHAPTER 1

Three Steps to Diagnosing Fibromyalgia

C hances are, you're reading this book because you suspect that either you or someone you love suffers from
fibromyalgia. But how can you be sure? Here are some
simple criteria you can use to perform a self-diagnosis:

FIRST TEST - CAUSES

Check any of the following potential causes
of fibromyalgia that apply to you:

____Poor, interrupted or non-refreshing sleep (1)
____Sleep apnea (2)
____Stress (1)
____Anxiety and/or panic disorders (2)
____Depression (2)
____Post-traumatic stress disorder (2)
____Bipolar disorder/manic-depression (2)
____Schizophrenia/other serious psychiatric disorders (2)
____Severe osteoarthritis/painful inflammatory diseases (2)
____Painful trauma such as a car accident (2)
____Restless legs syndrome (1)
____Hypermobility (double-jointed) (1)

Add up the numbers associated with each of the causes that you placed a check next to on the preceding page. If these add up to a sum greater than three, proceed to the next test.

SECOND TEST - SYMPTOMS

Have you noticed any of these symptoms?
Place a check mark next to those that apply to you:

___General pain, aches, stiffness

___Numbness

___Itching

___Feeling too cold or too hot

___Sensitivity to bright lights or loud noises

___Intense tastes or smells

___Skin that readily flushes

___Uncomfortable in a crowded environment

___Fatigue

___Confusion

Do your symptoms vary as the causes noted in the First Test intensify or improve? For example, do you tend to experience more pain and fatigue whenever your stress level is particularly high? Or, conversely, do you find you have more energy and suffer from less pain whenever you're able to get more sleep and avoid many of your normal stresses?

Do you have fibromyalgia?
If you have three or more points worth of causes and your symptoms vary with these causes, then you have fibromyalgia.

If you don't have fibromyalgia, there may be something else — a serious disease, perhaps, that's showing up in the form of pain and fatigue. It's precisely because of this possibility that I would never want anyone to follow the steps set forth in this book without first seeing a qualified health care practitioner to get a thorough examination. If you're suffering from a serious disease that has not yet been detected, there's really no time to waste in seeking out proper assessment and treatment.

THIRD TEST - OPTIONAL

This is entirely optional, but you may also want to ask your doctor for help in boosting your current dopamine levels. If, once you've succeeded in raising your dopamine levels, you notice that many or most of your symptoms subside, you can be 100 percent certain you have fibromyalgia.

There, that's it. With these three steps, you have the complete diagnostic criteria for fibromyalgia. They evolved entirely from my experiences with over a thousand patients who have the syndrome. For now, study the list of the causes and symptoms that apply to you, and begin noting how fluctuations in your particular causes directly relate to the intensity of the sensations, fatigue, and/or confusion associated with fibromyalgia.

CASE STUDY

MILDRED S.

Sixty-nine year old Mildred S. had been suffering with pain for about five years before seeing Dr. Dryland. Here's what she says about her experience.

MAJOR SYMPTOMS
"I ached all over. I hurt all the time. I couldn't do anything without hurting. I didn't really care what happened because I felt so bad all the time. That was happening for several years before I went to see him."

RESULTS
"His advice was good, definitely. After I went to see him I felt much better. I haven't felt like this for years!"

~

CHAPTER 2

What is Fibromyalgia?
Why Does it Hurt?

Fibromyalgia feels different to everyone. The common denominator in most cases is an elevated awareness of painful and other sensations throughout the body. Many of my fibromyalgia patients complain of feeling like they have the flu all the time, experience aches and pains throughout their bodies, are chronically tired, and often wake up feeling as if they have been in a car accident the day before. However, most people with fibromyalgia appear healthy. It is often difficult to identify a physical cause that explains the continued pain. Likewise, the blood tests for the usual pain-causing suspects such as rheumatoid arthritis, Lyme disease, or an underactive thyroid, amongst others, come back negative. The most frustrating and bewildering thing about fibromyalgia is that the symptoms people experience don't match the underlying physical causes – if a physical cause can even be found.

Although millions of people live with fibromyalgia, it is one of the most misunderstood and misdiagnosed illnesses of our time. When a person develops this disabling problem, it is natural to want to know what is wrong and how it can be cured. The prevailing wisdom in the medical community is that the pain originates in the fibers of the muscles, hence the name fibromyalgia – *fibro* meaning fiber and *myalgia* meaning muscle pain. If you've used my self-diagnosis test and found that you or someone you love has fibromyalgia, don't panic. Information is power. When patients come to my office with fibromyalgia symptoms, they are full of questions. In this chapter, I'll explain what fibromyalgia really is, address some of the most common misconceptions about it, and start you on the path to understanding and healing.

FIBROMYALGIA FACTS

How many people actually have fibromyalgia?
In most textbooks, it's estimated that up to 10 million of the more than 300 million people living in the United States have fibromyalgia. But there's a growing community of health care providers, including me, who believe this is a gross underestimate. If all the people who fit the correct definition of fibromyalgia were counted, I would guess the numbers would probably be closer to 30 million.

What is fibromyalgia?
Although fibromyalgia is often associated with painful muscles, it is not actually muscle pain. It is not a disease. You are not infected with anything. There is nothing broken or defective inside of you. In fact, it is just the opposite. Your mind is particularly effective at protecting you from dangers in the environment. Fibromyalgia is a matter of continually elevated adrenaline levels. They are increased to such a level that your ancient fight or flight response has been over-activated.

All animals have a stress response whenever danger is perceived. As we sense a threat, adrenaline (chemicals such as epinephrine and dopamine) is sent to our bodies to prepare us to either fight or run for our lives. If there really is a threat to your life, this automatic fight or flight response might be the one thing that helps you survive. This innate response has saved countless human lives over the course of human history, particularly in prehistoric times when life was more precarious. When rising levels of adrenaline activate the fight or flight response, some of our senses are actually more focused, allowing us to react to immediate danger. The fight or flight response also relies on dopamine, a chemical messenger, designed to keep us from feeling pain during the fight for our lives.

However, the fight or flight response was never designed to protect us from chronic non-life threatening dangers – the sort that besiege us regularly in our sped-up, hyper-stressed, modern day world.

The human mind cannot tell the difference between a physical threat and a psychological threat. Both will raise our adrenaline to such a level that our fight or flight response is initiated. Our nervous system, at least the part of it that responds to stress and danger, was meant to cycle – spiking in response to extraordinary stimuli, but generally remaining in perfect balance. In the absence of immediate danger, the normal rhythm calls for adrenaline to go up during the day and then down at night.

Individuals who experience increased adrenaline levels during the day without a substantial drop in those levels at night can develop fibromyalgia. Generally, people who suffer from fibromyalgia have to cope with too much adrenaline during the day followed by restless non-refreshing sleep at night. This combination often results in an adrenaline level that is continually elevated to such an extent that the fight or flight response is activated all the time, depleting valuable supplies of dopamine. An improperly activated fight or flight response is at the root of all the suffering that fibromyalgia causes.

Unfortunately, millions upon of people these days are not aware they have a fight or flight response. It is extremely harmful to be stuck in your fight or flight response as a consequence

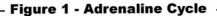

Figure 1 - Adrenaline Cycle

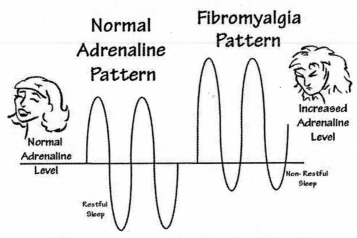

Normal adrenaline patterns go up during the day and then down at night for restful sleep. People with fibromyalgia experience too much adrenaline during the day and non-restful sleep at night.

of a bad marriage, a disagreeable job, or maybe even a bad back. It doesn't help that until recently, it wasn't understood that just such a situation might be what is triggering your fight or flight response and causing your fibromyalgia (Figure 1).

MYTH VS. FACT

Myth: Fibromyalgia is inflammation of the muscles.
The medical community has been telling patients for decades that fibromyalgia really amounts to "arthritis in the muscles." Initial studies did reveal abnormalities in the muscles in fibromyalgia patients, but the theories establishing a causal link were later disproved. Dr. Robert Simms of Boston University studied muscle energy metabolism in people with and without fibromyalgia. He found absolutely no differences or abnormalities in the muscles of fibromyalgia patients.[1] Once it was shown that there was no inflammation in the muscles, there was no longer any logical explanation for why these patients experienced pain.

The Simms study was completed in 1994, which was just about the time I finished medical school. Some of my professors and healthcare providers continued to insist that fibromyalgia was due to muscle inflammation despite this compelling evidence to the contrary. Because this and other misconceptions remain widespread, I would like to make several important points. If fibromyalgia was due to muscle inflammation, the pain should improve with the same strong anti-inflammatory medications used with other inflammatory diseases, such as rheumatoid arthritis. However, the strongest anti-inflammatory medication known today, prednisone, does very little for pain associated with fibromyalgia. Anti-inflammatory medication may help in cases where the patient has another painful condition as well.

Fact: Fibromyalgia does not damage your muscles.

If fibromyalgia were due to inflammation in the muscles, there would eventually be damage and destruction of the muscle tissue. We know this because in every other disease that involves inflammation, damage and destruction of tissue eventually results. The truth is that there is no inflammation or arthritis of the muscles associated with fibromyalgia. That is why your muscles look exactly the same despite years of pain. This is important to understand because I want to reassure you that your body is perfectly safe, which means that once you understand how fibromyalgia works, and can start to rein in your fight or flight response, you will have a perfectly healthy body waiting for you.

Myth: Only fibromyalgia patients have "Tender Points."

One of the classic methods for diagnosing fibromyalgia, is the identification of specific tender points across a person's body. These tender points are associated with areas where our ligaments and tendons insert into our bones. The presence or absence of these tender points does not necessarily confirm or dismiss a possible fibromyalgia diagnosis (Figure 2).

————— Figure 2 - Fibromyalgia Tender Points —————

Under the lower
sternomastoid muscle

Near the second
costochondral junction

2 cm distal to the
lateral epincondyle

At the prominence of
the greater trochanter

At the medial fat
pad of the knee

Insertion of the
suboccipital muscle

Mid upper
trapezius muscle

Origin of the
supraspinatus muscle

Upper outer quadrant
of the buttock

Fact: Everyone has tender points.

It's true that there are tender points that are associated with fibromyalgia. But we all are tender wherever our ligaments and tendons insert onto our bones. The difference is that most of us don't experience distress in those areas unless we do something like sleep on the floor or rub those areas particularly hard. It is only when our brains perceive amplified sensations that we become more aware of those tender spots, with pain signals being triggered by even just the lightest touch or slightest movement.

Any pressure applied to the classic tender points on a person with chronically elevated adrenaline levels will cause far more pain than if that person's adrenaline was cycling normally. In fact, this exaggeration effect applies to all the sensations we're able to perceive. This exaggeration effect can lead to heightened awareness. But it is also these altered sense perceptions that cause all of the suffering associated with fibromyalgia.

Myth: Fibromyalgia patients are either depressed or crazy.
During and after medical school, other professors and health care providers explained to me that patients with fibromyalgia symptoms were actually depressed or mentally unbalanced. There was a common belief that they were not actually in pain, and that fibromyalgia didn't really exist.

Fact: Fibromyalgia patients experience real pain.
The pain experienced by fibromyalgia patients is every bit as real as the pain suffered by any individual. Many patients with fibromyalgia, if not the majority, are not depressed or crazy. You do not have to be depressed to develop fibromyalgia. It is not unusual for people with fibromyalgia to subsequently experience depression as it can be such a life-altering illness. In addition, if you do happen to be depressed, it is still possible to improve your fibromyalgia symptoms without treating your depression.

THE FIBROMYALGIA/ ADRENALINE CONNECTION

*How do we know that fibromyalgia
is linked to increased adrenaline?*
There is currently an evolving body of evidence that supports my belief that fibromyalgia is associated with increased adrenaline rather than inflammation or arthritis.[2] When activated, the autonomic nervous system causes the adrenal glands to release adrenaline. In 1998, Dr. Satish Raj of Queen's University, Kingston, Ontario, Canada, studied the autonomic nervous system of fibromyalgia patients by causing them to faint (with the use of a tilt table) and then monitoring heart-rate variability. Dr. Raj found that the patients with fibromyalgia were over three times as likely to show abnormalities of the autonomic nervous as measured by an increase of adrenaline.[3]

What is RLS?

A correlation between restless legs syndrome (RLS) and fibromyalgia also provides evidence of increased adrenaline levels in fibromyalgia patients. RLS is described as an unpleasant feeling in the legs that results in uncontrollable twitching. Many patients with fibromyalgia have RLS. The RLS is thought to be related to increased adrenaline, specifically dopamine.[4] The association of RLS with fibromyalgia was proven by Dr. Muhammad Yunus.[5] I have certainly found this to be true in my own experience and with several hundred of my fibromyalgia patients.

The spontaneous jerking of the arms and legs of this syndrome usually happens when you are relaxing or trying to fall asleep. I believe this is the brain's way of literally trying to keep you from falling asleep because the "fight or flight response" has been activated. The brain is saying, "Wake up! It's not safe to fall asleep." If you have the restless legs syndrome associated with your fibromyalgia, you will likely notice that your restless jerks will begin to resolve as your fibromyalgia abates.

How can drugs for Parkinson's disease help fibromyalgia?

One of the most compelling pieces of evidence linking fibromyalgia to increased adrenaline levels is an abstract published by Dr. Andrew Holman and presented at the 2000 American College of Rheumatology annual convention. It detailed how he successfully treated fibromyalgia patients with pramipexole (Mirapex), a medication used for Parkinson's disease.

Mirapex helps regulate the adrenaline level and is also used to treat RLS. Dr. Holman found that high doses of Mirapex also greatly reduced the symptoms of fibromyalgia. Although these medications proved very hard to tolerate, the 50-60 percent of patients able to take Mirapex were cured of many of their fibromyalgia symptoms.[6]

For many of these patients, it was the first thing they had discovered that offered any relief. My work with hundreds of my own patients has duplicated these results. Although it is proven and accepted that patients with fibromyalgia have increased adrenaline, it is still unknown if this is the *cause* of fibromyalgia or simply the *effect* of having pain from fibromyalgia. Through my clinical observations, I have come to realize that it really is both. The fibromyalgia causes, by their very nature, will result in elevated adrenaline levels.

As the fight or flight response overreacts, the pain blocking substance dopamine becomes depleted, and you lose your ability to filter out sensations and begin to experience more pain and discomfort.

Additional testing will have to be done to prove this hypothesis, but I'm confident that human research will simply confirm the research already done on laboratory rats. As we burn through our limited supply of dopamine, we lose the protection that normally filters our full range of sensations.

Why does having an increased adrenaline level cause pain?

All sensations traveling into your brain are filtered in the limbic system, a small area in the base of your brain. It is the most important traffic center in your body. The limbic system actually involves several parts of your brain, but they all work closely together to play a vital role in interpreting the outside world for you. It also determines how you respond to what's happening in the outside world – which, among other things, means it controls your fight or flight response.

Normally, people do not feel all of their sensations. Someone under acute stress blocks many sensations. A person in chronic stress, with low dopamine levels from the overuse of their fight or flight response – loses their ability to filter out sensations and subsequently feels amplified sensations and pain (Figure 3).

Figure 3 - The Limbic System

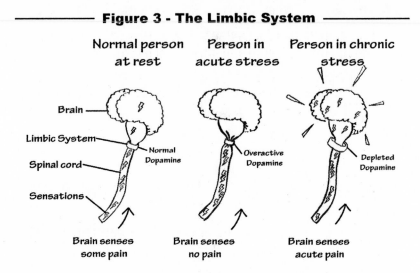

TRAFFIC CONTROL – THE LIMBIC SYSTEM

A bit of additional explanation is in order, since what's shown in this figure is key to your understanding fibromyalgia. Start with the assumption that all of our sensations are normally inhibited. That is, we never feel anything to the fullest extent. This is important because otherwise we'd be constantly aware of our clothes touching us and would be excruciatingly sensitive to any and all peripheral noise and light. You're not feeling your glasses or your socks all day long, but if you think about it, and focus on it you'll notice it. So all day long, you are filtering out the touch of your glasses, your socks, the hum of your refrigerator.

When we're under acute stress, the dopamine levels increase in this traffic center of the brain. This allows us to block even more sensations than normal. This increase allows us to respond to the external threat in a more focused way, and protects us from pain when we're facing life-threatening situations.

However, when the stress becomes chronic, the dopamine levels in this part of the brain eventually run low, leaving us to experience pain sensations even more fully than we normally do. So, in effect, whenever the fight or flight response is triggered too often or active for too long, we deplete our normal dopamine levels – leaving us with less than is necessary to inhibit sensations. We lose our ability to filter out the entire world and fibromyalgia is the result.

What proof is there that the brain perceives amplified sensations in fibromyalgia?

Tests with lab rats demonstrate the link between amplified sensory levels and fibromyalgia. A 1999 study by Altier and Stewart shows that when a rat first starts to experience acute stress – as a consequence of a forced swim, for example – it tends to be largely shielded from pain.[7] That's because the stress raises the rat's adrenaline level, specifically its dopamine level. This helps to block much of the pain the rat might normally experience (as the consequence of an injection, for instance).

People function in much the same way. Chances are, that you've heard stories of people who, when faced with incredibly stressful life-threatening situations such as a car crash, have managed to do some pretty incredible things without feeling pain. Those benefits are short-lived, however, and when the stress is chronic, the relief turns to intensified anguish.

Additional laboratory studies with rats have shown that chronic stress conditions are closely associated with increased pain sensations.[8] In fact, the stressed-out rats used in those studies continued to show a heightened response to painful stimuli for as long as a month after the chronic stress conditions were alleviated. Pain medications also proved to be less effective than normal with these chronically stressed rats. Similar results have since been reported in studies run at a variety of other labs.[9]

Many of these studies paid special attention to those areas of the rat brain where dopamine activity regularly intensifies in times of acute stress. This was found to be especially true in the part of the brain responsible for controlling the fight or flight response: the limbic system.

Here's how it works: although dopamine levels increased and clearly afforded the rats protection from pain during isolated instances of acute stress, under chronic stress it was discovered that the dopamine levels greatly decreased – not just to normal levels, but to less-than-normal levels. As a consequence, the rats felt more painful sensations as a result of using up their dopamine from staying in their fight or flight response too long.

The human nervous system is not one that fares well when suffering from fight or flight response fatigue. Instead, it was designed to perform vital services in brief, sporadic periods of acute danger, returning as quickly as possible to a state of restful calm. When we are stuck in a chronic fight or flight response, the brain effectively burns through its supply of pain-blocking dopamine in the limbic system.

Anyone with fibromyalgia can surely relate, because chronic physiological or psychological stress resulting in less than normal dopamine levels *is* fibromyalgia.

So what is actually happening in my body?

As hard as it is for most fibromyalgia patients to understand, nothing is actually being damaged in your body. The pain is so severe that most people quite naturally assume that something must be terribly wrong with the muscles and bones. However, even though the body remains perfectly fine and functional in every way, the pain associated with fibromyalgia is 100 percent genuine. And pain is just one of the many sensations that fibromyalgia serves to amplify.

THE PAIN THRESHOLD

How much does something hurt?

The point at which something hurts is our pain threshold. There is actually a threshold to feel anything, a sensation threshold. In the brain, particularly the limbic system, dopamine controls our sensation threshold. Dopamine blocks all sensations up to a certain point. Whenever a sensation is higher than the current level of dopamine, it will get through the limbic system and be sensed by the brain. Your current dopamine level determines your pain threshold (Figure 4).

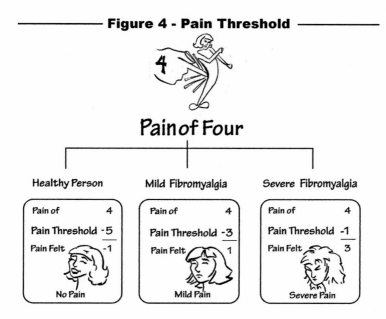

Figure 4 - Pain Threshold

Pain of Four

Healthy Person	Mild Fibromyalgia	Severe Fibromyalgia
Pain of 4	Pain of 4	Pain of 4
Pain Threshold -5	Pain Threshold -3	Pain Threshold -1
Pain Felt -1	Pain Felt 1	Pain Felt 3
No Pain	Mild Pain	Severe Pain

Most fibromyalgia patients also experience numbness, itching, problems with being too hot or too cold. Some even find it difficult to be in a crowded environment. Every sense perception the human body experiences is intensified. Whenever your adrenaline fails to cycle properly, you can expect to experience an overwhelming sense of fatigue, attended by a confused feeling that some call "fibro fog."

Most fibromyalgia patients also experience altered and/or overactive sensations such as intensified tastes and smells, and intolerance to bright lights or loud noises (Figure 5).

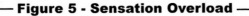

Figure 5 - Sensation Overload

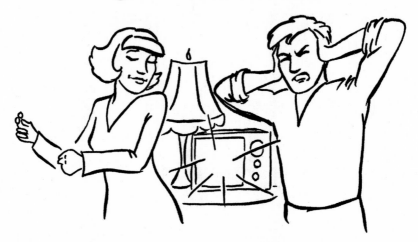

Normal Sensations   Overactive Sensations

Can I be tested to see if I have an activated fight or flight response?

Tests exist to measure adrenaline levels, but they're usually unnecessary. Heart rate variability monitoring is available through most cardiologists. Beyond that, there are many other tests of brain activity, including PET scans.

I don't recommend these tests, primarily for two reasons. The first is that fibromyalgia is reasonably straightforward to diagnose (see Chapter 1), making it unnecessary to check your adrenaline level (assuming you're confident in the competence of your health care practitioner). My second reservation is that I'd prefer that people first attempt to heal themselves once they've been able to develop a suitable plan. This book will allow you to do just that. Otherwise, my fear is that your fibromyalgia will be treated as a disease, which is inappropriate for reasons I'll explain later.

If it's all so simple, why hasn't the medical community not been able to figure it out?

The answer here is as complicated as medicine itself. Certainly, I wouldn't want to suggest that physicians don't care about this condition or the patients that have it. The fact is that many physicians and researchers take these patients quite seriously. But even though the incidence of fibromyalgia is quite common, its nature is rather uncommon. That is, it's rare that such suffering can result from nothing more than a slight alteration of a normal function in the human mind. Depression, perhaps, is somewhat analogous. Irritable bowel syndrome is probably even more akin to fibromyalgia.

Health care providers also want to understand what it is they're trying to treat. Fibromyalgia is not only poorly understood, but can also be quite frustrating to treat. That is, it's not the sort of thing that can typically be diagnosed and treated in the 10-15 minutes usually allocated to each patient visit. Unfortunately, this has led many in the health care community to shy away from treating fibromyalgia. Worse yet, some doctors go so far as to deny that fibromyalgia even exists.

Health care providers also want to understand what it is they're trying to treat. Fibromyalgia is not only poorly understood, but can also be quite frustrating to treat.

Because of my own experience with fibromyalgia patients and my familiarity with the current research in this area, it's been clear to me for some time that fibromyalgia has never been a disease, but rather a problem with the normal function of the human mind. Once I determined the underlying causes, I was also able to develop an easy-to-follow diagnostic criteria. And with that, I've been able to help patients figure out their own particular causes and choose the remedy that's right for them from four basic choices:

1) **Work on the causes.**

2) **Take suitable prescribed medications.**

3) **Partake in treatments that provide comfort, such as heat or massage.**

4) **Regulate adrenaline levels through medication.**

Please remember that it is never too late to treat your fibromyalgia. Whether you've suffered through decades of pain or just six months of it, the lessons in this book should hold true for you, serving as your definitive guide to what fibromyalgia is and what you can do about it.

I welcome you to learn all you can so you can choose the path to recovery that's best for you. The time for that is now. Because while it's never too late to get your life back, you're probably thinking that it can't happen soon enough.

CASE STUDY
DIANA F.

Registered Nurse Diana F. was working at a hospital when her symptoms became severe. Here's what she has to say about her experience.

MAJOR SYMPTOMS

"I can go back a very long way that I have had symptoms, but when it really got bad was in 1989. I'm a nurse, an RN. I was pushing a patient on a gurney up a ramp when I twisted my knee. I ended up having arthroscopy. I went back to work after the first one, but then it didn't get better, my knee didn't get better. I kept having more symptoms."

RESULTS

"I waited several months to see Dr. Dryland. When I got to see him the very first thing he said to me was, 'Has anybody ever told you what causes fibromyalgia?' I said no. He said, 'This is what causes it...' and told me all about it. Now it's like a difference between night and day. He was the first person ever who gave me some hope and also who just plain understood because he suffered from it himself and he knows the horror it is."

~

CHAPTER 3

Unveiling the Causes of Fibromyalgia

O ver the course of this chapter, I'll cover what causes fibromyalgia, as well as what doesn't cause it. In addition, I'll explain how these causes feed into the vicious cycle of fibromyalgia. Understanding this cycle is the key to attaining relief for most patients, especially in the most severe cases of fibromyalgia, where people have lost hope of ever getting better. You may not have all of these causes as the list is quite long.

FIBROMYALGIA CAUSES

- Poor, interrupted or non-refreshing sleep
- Sleep apnea (breathing irregularities while sleeping)
- Stress
- Anxiety and panic disorders
- Depression
- Post-traumatic stress disorder
- Bipolar disorder/manic-depression
- Schizophrenia or other serious psychiatric disorders
- Severe osteoarthritis or painful inflammatory diseases
- Painful trauma, such as a car accident
- Restless legs syndrome
- Hypermobility (double-jointed)

Poor, interrupted, or non-refreshing sleep

Sleep has five basic stages, Stages 1 through 4 and then REM (or dream sleep). Contrary to popular belief, it is those stages right before our dream or REM sleep, Stages 3 and 4, where we gain most of our refreshment and manage to restore our bodies for another day.

In 1974, Dr. Harvey Moldofsky published a landmark study that showed how pain could be induced by interrupting Stages 3 and 4 of sleep. Dr. Moldofsky hired healthy students aged 19-25 and deprived six of them of Stage 4 sleep and seven of them of REM sleep. This was done for three nights running. The subjects whose Stage 4 sleep had been interrupted began showing signs of fibromyalgia. This wasn't the case for the subjects who had been denied REM sleep. In addition, the students who had been deprived of their Stage 4 sleep began to experience overwhelming tiredness, loss of appetite, and one even suffered from nausea and diarrhea. Once sleep was restored to normal for these subjects, all of their fibromyalgia symptoms disappeared.[1]

I have had several fibromyalgia patients referred to me whose sleep patterns had already been analyzed. Their studies showed that they were getting very little Stage 3 sleep and virtually no Stage 4 sleep. In other words, their sleep patterns closely approximated the conditions Dr. Moldofsky created for his sleep study when he was actually trying to induce fibromyalgia in his patients.

Another study that reinforces what Dr. Moldofsky found was mounted by Dr. Glenn Affleck at the University of Connecticut, who set out to analyze the sleep patterns of 50 women with fibromyalgia. He discovered that whenever any of these women suffered a poor night of sleep, it was almost invariably followed by a day of intensified pain.[2]

Sleep apnea

Sleep apnea is an obstruction of breathing or even a complete cessation of breathing during sleep. The body then awakens itself out of deep sleep to begin breathing again. This is all happening unconsciously. Sleep apnea is one of the hidden causes of fibromyalgia, especially for men. A test conducted by Dr. K. May, a rheumatologist at the Fitzsimons Army Medical Center, confirms this. In the test, subjects were first screened with a questionnaire that asked about their sleep apnea symptoms. Those that met Dr. May's criteria were then studied in a sleep lab, where she found that 44 percent of the male subjects did indeed suffer from sleep apnea. Only 2.2 percent of the female patients, on the other hand, were found to have sleep apnea.[3]

Most people with sleep apnea don't realize it until they're diagnosed. What they do know, however, is that they regularly wake up very tired, possibly with a headache, and that they sometimes even awaken in pain or a state of confusion. These people also have a tendency to gain weight, suffer from high blood pressure, and often contend with a host of other serious health problems.

Still, people can carry on like this for years — but generally not without disturbing their loved ones. Often, in fact, the spouse or some other family member will report that they have regularly observed severe snoring or even periods of up to 30 seconds where no breathing at all has occurred (it's these episodes that are referred to as "apneas").

I regularly ask each fibromyalgia patient as well as their spouse and other family members to see if they've noted any of these symptoms. Many will joke and say, "Yup, I just wait for him to start breathing again. Sometimes it's scary." That's right, and it's scary for your body too. There's nothing like nearly dying every night to drive your adrenaline levels right off the chart.

And that's exactly how your body reacts whenever your oxygen level plunges because you've stopped breathing. So what happens then? Your body literally snaps out of Stage 3 or 4 sleep in order to start breathing again. This is our basic mammalian reflex to what's perceived as suffocation. For people with undiagnosed sleep apnea, this can happen hundreds of times each night! This amounts to an adrenaline rush all night long. So it's no wonder that you then wake up tired, confused and in pain.

Altogether, I have found that approximately five percent of my fibromyalgia patients have been laboring for years with undiagnosed sleep apnea. That percentage is higher for men, as well as for anyone who's overweight.

Stress
It probably will come as no surprise that stress is one of the most common causes of fibromyalgia. In fact, it rates with poor sleep as one of the leading causes. And, of course, it only makes sense that if you happen to be stressed about something, your adrenaline levels are almost certain to go up.

That's not all either, since stress and anxiety also typically cause our blood pressure and pulse rates to rise. The body also makes other adjustments to stress, most of which are unhealthy for you in the long run. Stress is often associated with heart disease, ulcers and deficiencies in your immune system. And what triggers all of these things? Rising adrenaline levels.

Still, for most people stress seems unavoidable. If you're one such person, don't lose hope. As we will see, you don't need to eliminate all of your stress to treat your fibromyalgia.

Anxiety and panic disorders
People who suffer from a combination of chronic anxiety and panic disorders generally face more serious consequences than do those who simply have to deal with high levels of stress. Both anxiety and panic disorders have a well-documented association with increased levels of adrenaline. How can you tell the difference between the two? Typically, panic attacks involve the sudden onset of intense fear or terror.

Generalized anxiety disorder, on the other hand, is more constant, characterized by chronically high levels of worry and anxiety that are difficult to control and typically result in significant distress and impairment.

In addition to the obvious psychological strain, people who suffer from these mental disorders also tend to manifest physical symptoms. Which is to say, they can develop fibromyalgia.

As already observed in Chapter 2, whenever you find yourself in continual fight or flight mode, you are apt to sense things in your body you were never meant to. Many patients suffering from panic disorder experience intense chest pain despite having no obvious heart problems. What's most likely happening is that the panic disorder has left the patient effectively stuck in fight or flight mode, with chronically elevated adrenaline levels, intensifying awareness of pain in the area of the chest where connective tissues come together. In fact, fibromyalgia is often first detected in patients who initially sought medical attention for what they thought to be heart attacks.[4]

Unfortunately, after some of these patients are told there's actually nothing wrong with their hearts, they may start to think they're crazy and over-reacting. However, as we are learning, the pain they're experiencing is 100 percent genuine. These patients feel the connective tissue in their chest more than normal because they're stuck in their fight or flight response and have depleted their dopamine. During the panic attack, they further exhaust their dopamine supply and subsequently feel like they are having a heart attack.

Depression

Depression is a broad area that can include intense depression, a more temporary response to grief, chronic depressed mood (dysthmia), and what has been termed as 'normal' depression. It's true that depression is entirely normal and is woven into each person's lifelong development, surfacing periodically in response to all manner of life events. Although the exact brain chemistry has yet to be determined, dopamine is certainly believed to play a role.

As a human being, you almost certainly can remember a time when you were depressed and so can probably recall how you experienced excessive worry or anxiety during that time, along with altered moods, sleep difficulties, and/or fatigue.

I believe that when we're depressed, our brain acts on the assumption that something is wrong and compensates by raising adrenaline levels. Certainly if you're chronically depressed, your fight or flight response is already overactive. So whenever anything else happens that's apt to cause your adrenaline not to cycle properly, it probably will have an exaggerated effect — and could easily lead to fibromyalgia.

Post-Traumatic Stress Disorder (PTSD)

Generally speaking, PTSD applies to any stress that remains long after the trauma that caused it has receded into history. Post-Traumatic Stress Disorder is a very common cause of fibromyalgia — so much so, in fact, that many in the medical community operated under the assumption that all patients with fibromyalgia had been abused or had extreme trauma at some point. This, of course, is simply not true.

Patients with PTSD often describe the intense adrenaline rushes they get whenever they're having a flashback. It is a tragedy that people who have experienced a severe trauma are faced with reliving it over and over and over again. The body actually experiences the trauma anew, using up dopamine with each succeeding flashback. These flashbacks can be triggered at any time by thoughts, discussions, random events that strike some familiar chord, or even just the mere anticipation of the anniversary of the event in question.

And that's not all. You don't even have to be experiencing flashbacks to have your PTSD trigger fibromyalgia. Many patients have had prolonged traumatic experiences where they have felt trapped for months or years in an abusive situation (be it sexual, emotional or physical). PTSD can also result from a bad childhood, marriage, or relationship; or a prolonged stressful situation in the face of extreme poverty, famine, crime, or some other difficult living circumstance. Whenever we experience anything of the sort for an extended period of time, our bodies become accustomed to operating in habitual fight or flight mode.

Even after escaping such terrible circumstances and leaving them far behind, the residual effect is having a fight or flight response that is on a hair-trigger. I've tended to many patients who've insisted they've managed to put their PTSD and the associated flashback episodes behind them through years of therapy. Unfortunately, even after the flashbacks stop, the hypersensitive fight or flight response often remains.

Bipolar Disorder (Manic Depression)

In my opinion, bipolar disorder is one of the hardest causes to treat. However, I also want to emphasize that it can be successfully treated. Bipolar disorder is a serious mental illness in which manic episodes are interspersed within a more general condition of depression. Manic episodes are characterized by exceptionally elevated or irritable moods accompanied by unusually high self-esteem, a reduced need for sleep, bursts of chattiness, racing thoughts, and/or unrestrained involvement in pleasurable activities with long-term consequences (including gambling, shopping sprees and dangerous sexual activity). These manic episodes can often have terrible consequences.

However, there are people with bipolar disorder who have enjoyed tremendous success, including world leaders, respected thinkers, and famous artists. But for all their success, many of these people probably also kick their legs at night, sleep poorly, and ache all the time. Which is to say they may certainly have fibromyalgia.

It is interesting to note that the adrenaline curve for a bipolar patient is similar to a non-bipolar patient who has fibromyalgia. That means that the bipolar person's adrenaline levels, although almost certainly too high when they're manic, in all likelihood cycles back to "normal" whenever they feel depressed. Their adrenaline level probably never goes below normal, but drops to something below their greatly elevated manic level. Whenever patients with bipolar disorder are treated with medications to normalize their adrenaline level there's a good chance they'll start to feel very depressed.

Another point worth noting is that there actually are two different forms of bipolar disorder:

Bipolar I – a person with documented manic episodes.

Bipolar II – a person who suffers from major depression, but with much milder mania.

As you might suspect, it's easier to help people with the latter version gain control of their fibromyalgia. It's also possible with Bipolar I, but much more difficult.

Schizophrenia (and other serious mental illnesses)
It is beyond the scope of this book to delve into these problems. Suffice it to say that although much of the brain chemistry related to serious mental illness remains a mystery, it is believed to be related to adrenaline levels. The drugs used to treat Schizophrenia, called neuroleptics, work by "tranquilizing" the subject, likely by lowering the adrenaline level among other things.

Osteoarthritis (wear and tear), Lupus, Rheumatoid Arthritis, and other inflammatory or painful diseases
Osteoarthritis, lupus, rheumatoid arthritis and other inflammatory diseases each have one thing in common: they all cause pain. And, more often than not, rheumatologists are the physicians people turn to for relief.

As you probably already know, whenever we're in pain, our blood pressure and pulse rise. Adrenaline plays an important role in this. Apart from suffocating nightly as a consequence of sleep apnea, there's nothing that's better at getting the attention of your fight or flight response than pain. Unfortunately, it's this pain that can end up triggering fibromyalgia. Most patients then ask, "But I thought you said fibromyalgia is pain?"

Yes, but there's a difference between the pain that causes fibromyalgia and that which results from fibromyalgia.

We'll explore this confusing distinction in the next chapter.

For reasons that probably are starting to sound familiar to you, people who suffer with painful arthritis in their joints (lupus, for example) are halfway to getting fibromyalgia as well. That's because with their already elevated adrenaline levels (raised in response to the arthritic pain), these people also have a fight or flight response that's on a hair-trigger. A bout of depression or a poor night's sleep might be all it takes to kick the adrenaline system into chronic overdrive. What this amounts to, unfortunately, is that the margin of safety for patients who already suffer with painful conditions is ever so slim. Any further dopamine depletion will result in fibromyalgia.

Painful trauma from a particular incident
Any painful trauma, it turns out, can result in elevated adrenaline levels. Although this point is currently debated within the medical community, I maintain that physical trauma almost certainly causes fibromyalgia as well. That's because I've treated many patients who were able to handle poor sleep or stress just fine until such time as they suffered some sort of physical trauma. Maybe they slipped and fell at work, or perhaps they were involved in a car accident. The list of possibilities is endless.

The important point here is that just about anything that causes pain will result in higher adrenaline levels. The longer the duration of that pain and the more intense its severity, the greater the chance it will end up raising your adrenaline to such a level that your fight or flight mechanism is activated. Another painful trauma is all the more likely to cause fibromyalgia if you already are having problems with stress, depression or sleep.

It works the other way as well. That is, a person who is largely pain-free could have a car accident that suddenly changes everything. That person's adrenaline level immediately goes up while at the same time their margin of safety narrows. Then matters are compounded as more pain, poor sleep, depression, and/or stress follows. Before long, our previously perfectly healthy person is in a downward spiral, which within a few short months could lead to severe fibromyalgia.

Hypermobility Syndrome (double jointed)

People with lax or loose joints often complain of pain similar to fibromyalgia. These pains may simply stem from the trauma their loose joints regularly experience. However, together with a colleague, Dr. Holman, I've found hypermobile joints to be a major contributing cause of fibromyalgia. Which is to say that anyone who is double-jointed is likely to get fibromyalgia if they also have any of the other causes noted in this section.

Restless Legs Syndrome

The uncomfortable and uncontrollable jerking leg and arm motion that afflicts many fibromyalgia sufferers is directly related to high adrenaline levels.

At first, it may appear to be more a symptom than a cause of fibromyalgia. And in most cases, that's true. However, it takes much less adrenaline than is characteristic of fibromyalgia to initiate the restless legs syndrome. Also, there are many patients with restless legs and arms who do not have fibromyalgia.

However, once people with the restless legs syndrome acquire one or more of the other causes of fibromyalgia listed here, the restless legs syndrome can start to act as a contributing cause in its own right. Also, in those cases where a diagnosis of fibromyalgia is not entirely certain, the presence of restless legs tends to alleviate any doubts.

IF I DON'T HAVE ANY OF THE CAUSES, CAN I STILL HAVE FIBROMYALGIA?

If you don't have any of the causes listed above, you don't have fibromyalgia. See your health care provider to find out what's really at the root of your symptoms. Instances where patients think they may have fibromyalgia but insist they have none of the typical causes are extremely rare – perhaps 1 in 1000. And this leaves us with only three possibilities:

1) You may have one of the causes of fibromyalgia that's difficult for you to detect, such as lupus or sleep apnea. I have often found fibromyalgia to be the symptom that ultimately leads to a diagnosis of lupus.

2) There may be something else – a serious disease, perhaps, that's showing up in the form of pain and fatigue. It's precisely because of this possibility that I would never want anyone to follow the steps set forth in this book without first seeing a qualified health care practitioner to get a thorough examination. If you're suffering from a serious disease that has not yet been detected, there's really no time to waste in seeking out proper assessment and treatment.

3) Something may be interfering with your ability to properly assess what your body is experiencing. For example, if you have Post-Traumatic Stress Disorder, you may not have healed as

thoroughly as you think you have. That is, you may think you've put it all behind you, but your adrenaline system is still inclined to elevate readily. In much the same way, many people with Type A personalities get to a point in their lives where they think they've learned how to handle their stress appropriately. But, in fact, their adrenaline systems may still be operating according to old conditioning.

Are you one of these people? Pause a moment to ask yourself: Do you feel as though your adrenaline level is often too high? Do you feel on edge? Are you easily startled? Do you tend to show anger or defensiveness more than those around you? Have you ever experienced road rage? Do your legs jerk at night? Do you have trouble sleeping?

These are important questions, because if none of the psychological causes associated with fibromyalgia apply to you, there may be a previously undetected disease that lies at the root of your fibromyalgia-like symptoms — and that disease may require the immediate attention of a qualified health care provider.

FIBROMYALGIA MISCONCEPTIONS

The multitude of misconceptions regarding the causes of fibromyalgia stem from the decades when very little was known about fibromyalgia. Generally speaking, they fall into three basic categories.

1) *The fibromyalgia blame game.*
Being overweight does not cause fibromyalgia. It's true that many people gain weight when their adrenaline is cycling improperly. You may have noticed a slow but steady weight gain since you have had fibromyalgia. Fortunately, if your weight gain is from your fibromyalgia, things should improve as you treat your fibromyalgia, even if you make no other changes with diet and

exercise. But simply having extra pounds on your frame will not cause fibromyalgia unless you are also depressed and losing sleep over your weight. And remember, a stressful crash diet and exercise program is likely to make your fibromyalgia much worse.

It's also wrong to blame fibromyalgia on a lack of exercise. With mild cases of fibromyalgia, it's true that some exercise can help people feel better and more energetic. But with more severe cases of fibromyalgia, strenuous exercise is actually likely to make things much worse.

That's because fibromyalgia causes your brain to perceive amplified sensations — meaning that even the slight pulls and normal aches that come with modest exercise can lead to tremendous suffering.

Another popular misconception is that fibromyalgia is in some way related to certain foods. Mind you, if you already are struggling with adrenaline levels that are exceptionally high, it's clearly not a good idea to down a cup of coffee or a sugary snack just prior to retiring for the evening. And many people who suffer from fibromyalgia feel worse if they eat simple carbohydrates, that is, lots of sugar. This is likely due to the sugar high that temporarily raises your adrenaline. Apart from that, I'm afraid all the low-fat and low-carb diets in the world aren't likely to have much of an effect on your fibromyalgia.

Other misconceptions hold that the roots of fibromyalgia are to be found in your posture, your choice of clothes, your spouse, your furniture, your level of education, your community, your exposure to chemical effluents, your genetics, the amount of Candida in your gut, and any number of other things. But you can strike all such notions off your list unless they somehow cause your adrenaline levels to rise by inducing pain, interrupting your sleep, causing depression or stressing you out.

2) Problems related to increased adrenaline levels but not associated with fibromyalgia.

Increased levels of adrenaline can do much more than cause confusion, fatigue, and amplified sensations. Whenever our adrenaline is up, we start to feel edgy, we sweat more, our skin flushes more readily, and our immune systems function poorly. Chronic stress, moreover, can lead to heart disease, peptic ulcers and many other serious or life-threatening health problems. Although fibromyalgia results from increased adrenaline, there are many other problems that result from increased adrenaline besides pain, fatigue, and confusion.

3) You are somehow responsible for fibromyalgia.

Let me state this as clearly as I possibly can: *You did nothing to cause your fibromyalgia.* The pain is not your fault. You did not choose to have fibromyalgia, nor did you exercise any choice (conscious, unconscious or otherwise) in activating your fight or flight response. Your genetic programming flipped that switch for you automatically.

But before you start cursing your genetic makeup, just remember that we have our innate fight or flight response to thank for our very existence as a human species. A few thousand years ago, the fight or flight response may have made you a hero. Today, though, your fight or flight response can cause you much more harm than good — unless you spend much of your life on the battlefield where actions based on your quickened impulses are entirely appropriate (and necessary to ensure your survival).

Most of us, though, don't live our lives on battlefields. So what do your quickened impulses do for you when your boss yells at you? If you take action on the basis of those impulses, you'll probably get fired. So, more likely, you and your elevated adrenaline levels will probably have no choice but to sit and stew in your cubicle — while you continue to get more and more angry, stressed, and depressed. And if you have fibromyalgia, your symptoms will only worsen as your adrenaline level continues to climb. Chances are, if you have fibromyalgia you've been experiencing something very much along these lines for years now. And no wonder — this is a very familiar phenomenon I call the "the vicious cycle of fibromyalgia."

THE VICIOUS CYCLE OF FIBROMYALGIA

How common is this cycle? Just think of all the people you know who seem to be doing just fine in spite of the occasional bout of depression or period of poor sleep until they have their first baby. Then, in many cases, their lives start coming undone. After a few weeks of euphoria, poor sleep and stress begin to take their toll.

———— Figure 6 - Fibromyalgia Cycle ————

Once increased adrenaline levels trigger fibromyalgia, the vicious cycle begins (Figure 6). That is, with the pain, confusion, and fatigue of fibromyalgia comes additional stress, worse sleep and deeper depression — all of which leads to even higher adrenaline

41

levels and the continued depletion of your dopamine levels. This spiral can continue indefinitely, leading in many cases to devastating consequences and severe fibromyalgia.

For some people the initial event responsible for triggering the vicious cycle may have occurred years — or even decades — earlier. Thus, while the event itself may be all but forgotten, its repercussions remain just as vivid as ever.

My own experience with patients suggests that people tend to enter the fibromyalgia cycle anywhere from a few months to 2-3 years after the traumatic event itself has taken place. At times it can be hard to even figure out what that triggering event must have been. Remember, after all, that the potential sources for stress, pain, and sleep disruption are innumerable.

In terms of isolating the cause responsible for your case of fibromyalgia, look back at the events that took place in your life anywhere from a few months to 2-3 years prior to when you first noticed symptoms of fibromyalgia. It could be that the experience you end up identifying as the triggering event was just simply the last in an already long list of potential causes. That is, you may end up concluding that it was the news of your son's divorce that ultimately pushed you over the top. But would that news have affected you in the same way had you not already suffered through a stressful childhood and a disastrous divorce yourself?

The stories of what leads to fibromyalgia are as unique as the people who tell them. The one thing that's common to virtually every one of these accounts is that once the fibromyalgia cycle gets initiated, things start going downhill rapidly.

People who have fibromyalgia soon learn that they are more prone to many of the conditions listed at the beginning of this chapter, each of which only serves to compound the suffering and perpetuate the fibromyalgia cycle. It's in this way that the cycle can continue unbroken for years, or even for the rest of your life.

Figure 7 - What Keeps You Trapped

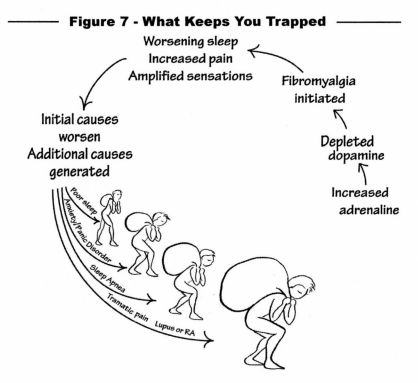

Worsening sleep
Increased pain
Amplified sensations

Fibromyalgia
initiated

Initial causes
worsen
Additional causes
generated

Depleted
dopamine

Increased
adrenaline

Poor sleep
Anxiety/Panic Disorder
Sleep Apnea
Tramatic pain
Lupus or RA

When the fibromyalgia cycle gets initiated, things start going downhill rapidly. The key to finding relief is to understand what keeps you trapped in the cycle (Figure 7). Only then can you take the steps required to break the fibromyalgia cycle and start reclaiming your life.

CASE STUDY

VICKY G.

Fifty-eight year old Vicky G. had her fibromyalgia symptoms for 18 years before she started working with Dr. Dryland. Here's what she has to say about her experience.

MAJOR SYMPTOMS

"I had been suffering with it for years. Everybody kept telling me that it was osteoarthritis. But then the symptoms kept getting worse and worse and my hands kept getting stiffer, and I kept having this horrendous pain in my neck and my ankles. I kept getting the pain and I kept going to the doctors telling them I had this pain. They told me there was nothing wrong with me."

RESULTS

"I didn't know anything about fibromyalgia. After Dr. Dryland told me about the causes of fibromyalgia I started picking up that I probably have suffered with this longer than the osteoarthritis. All my life I've been under stress. Now I've figured out a way to make it better. Dr. Dryland saved my life!"

~

CHAPTER 4

What Will Fibromyalgia Do to Me?

Now that you know what fibromyalgia is, let's take a closer look at what it can, and cannot, do to you. I want to reiterate that all of the discomfort and pain you experience when you're in the throes of fibromyalgia is 100 percent real. No matter what anybody else thinks, you're not crazy. And you're not a victim of bad luck or a person who suddenly became far more injury-prone. You're simply noticing sensations that weren't obvious to you before. And even the sensations that were evident before are intensified in a deeply unsettling way.

COMMON QUESTIONS

How does fibromyalgia harm my body?

As I explained in Chapter 2, fibromyalgia will not damage your body! Fibromyalgia greatly intensifies normal pain signals that you wouldn't otherwise notice. Once your fight or flight response has been engaged for an extended period, you need only touch those areas lightly or move your body ever so slightly to experience tremendous pain.

And yet, the only thing that's really changed physically is that your central nervous system has shifted into a higher gear and you have lost the ability to filter out sensations because of your depleted dopamine levels.

Besides pains, aches, and stiffness, these sensations can include uncomfortable numbness, tingling, itching, periods where you're either too hot or too cold, skin flushing, an altered sense of taste and smell, discomfort in crowds, an intolerance to bright lights and certain visual patterns, and loud noises. Fatigue and confusion are also quite common whenever your adrenaline isn't cycling properly. Fortunately, as they relate to your fibromyalgia, these symptoms will disappear as you heal your body.

Do the classic fibromyalgia "tender points" provide an accurate diagnosis?

As I briefly discussed in Chapter 2, every single human being has the classic "fibromyalgia tender points" — along with many others as well. According to current diagnostic criteria set by the American College of Rheumatology, patients with the history of widespread pain and who report pain in 11 of the 18 tender points shown in Figure 7, are diagnosed to have fibromyalgia. To understand why these areas are called "tender points", ask a friend or family member to let you apply light pressure to one of these spots on their body.

Next, apply similar pressure just a few inches away from that tender point. Repeat the same test in as many other areas as is necessary to satisfy your curiosity (or exhaust the patience of your volunteer test subject). You'll find that your friend or family member consistently reports more sensitivity at the indicated tender points than anywhere else. This goes to show that we all have tender points — fibromyalgia or otherwise.

—————— **Figure 7 - Fibromyalgia Tender Points** ——————

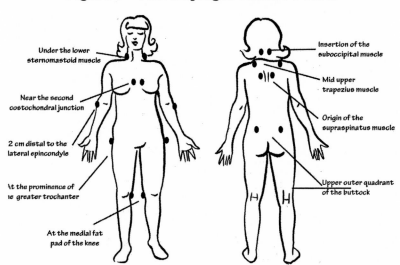

This is one of the reasons why I think it's a mistake to base a fibromyalgia diagnosis solely on the strength of reported pain in the indicated trigger points. Another problem with the classic diagnostic criteria is that only 80 percent of the people suffering from fibromyalgia — at most — experience exceptional pain in their tender points. So the current accepted diagnostic criteria totally misses people who may have been spared exceptional pain, but who still have to cope with the amplified sensations or overwhelming fatigue of a fight or flight response kicked into overdrive.

I've had many patients referred to me who initially reported nothing more than numbness or tingling. But in many of these cases, with reference to the criteria described in the Chapter 1, I was able to quickly determine that the reported sensations actually were the result of fibromyalgia. More often than not, these patients had been searching for answers for years — through countless MRI scans, neurological assessments, surgeries to repair entrapped nerves, and various other tests and procedures. A few of these folks had given up all hope of ever learning what was wrong with them. And in every one of these cases, fibromyalgia had already been eliminated as a possibility simply because these were people who were not reporting pain in their tender points.

Why do so many people with fibromyalgia have tight knots in their muscles?

Figure 8 - Pain of Ten

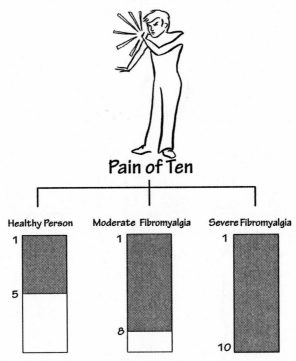

Pain of Ten

With a painful touch of 10, all of our pain receptors are activated. A person with a normal level of dopamine (a pain threshold of 5) will feel a pain of 5 as dopamine blocks half of the stimulus (Figure 8). A moderate fibromyalgia sufferer with a pain threshold of 2 will feel unbearable pain of 8, and a severe fibromyalgia sufferer with a pain threshold of 0 will feel a suicidal pain of 10. The lower your dopamine level the more knots you will notice and the more painful they will be.

50

We all sustain tight muscle knots, pulls, strains, tears, and stiffness as a consequence of engaging in a wide array of activities. But for most of us, those knots, pulls, strains or tears have to be fairly serious before we even take note of them. That's to say, we always have mildly painful areas throughout our bodies. It's just that we're generally not aware of those sensations, as normal levels of dopamine block most of these in the limbic system. Once we lose this filter, every muscle knot and strain is readily apparent.

With severe fibromyalgia, the pain can be so intense that most people can't imagine it stems from nothing more than a muscle knot. And this is precisely why most health care providers, family members, and fibromyalgia patients have such a hard time believing that nothing more serious is wrong with their bodies.

This tends to greatly complicate the diagnosis. The patients themselves suspect that something has gone terribly wrong with their bodies. Their family members are often unsympathetic because, to their eye, the person who claims to be suffering looks perfectly normal. Health care providers, meanwhile, spend much of their time looking for more serious problems, simply because it seems unlikely that someone could possibly be suffering so much from a muscle knot. As a consequence, lab tests, CT scans, and exploratory surgeries often follow.

As indicated in the final part of Figure 8, a fibromyalgia patient with a threshold of "0" will feel every single muscle knot, pull or strain they ever get. And a tight muscle knot of severity 10 will cause suffering that truly goes off the charts.

When people feel pain to this severity, visits to the local emergency room are common. But unfortunately, this rarely leads to relief while it often manages to deepen the frustration and confusion the fibromyalgia sufferer already feels. Typically, the emergency room doctor on duty will be unable to either provide relief or an explanation – and neither will the surgeon. Following a few tests, the patient will often be told that absolutely nothing is wrong since all test results look perfectly normal.

But that doesn't make the person with fibromyalgia feel any better. It's possible that their suffering is so great that they may not even be able to go back to work. They may attempt to exercise and end up aggravating the situation even more. And so the vicious cycle of fibromyalgia will continue as dopamine is further depleted. When an even more intense muscle knot appears, it is even more painful then the one before. It's no wonder people can start to lose all hope.

Why do even clothes sometimes feel uncomfortable?

Many patients have told me that certain clothes make them extremely uncomfortable. Certain fabrics as well seem to be particularly problematic. But what is it that's really at the root of this irritation? Often, it turns out to be nothing more serious than the friction created by rubbing up against a loose thread, the hem on their pants, or the manufacturer's tag at the back of their neck. The people making these complaints are folks who have worn clothes all their lives without any similar problems. It's just that with their fight or flight response working overtime, all of their normal sensations are now perceived as amplified.

Of course, with sensations like these, it's only natural that people want to get answers and relief as quickly as possible. This explains why many people with fibromyalgia end up going to so many different health care providers searching for answers and finding none. It's not just the misery that fibromyalgia causes either, because once you lose your ability to filter sensations, virtually every other malady – be it an allergy, lower back pain, endometriosis, a rash, the flu, or carpal tunnel syndrome will be exaggerated. And the hypersensitivity that's the signature of fibromyalgia also means that anything and everything that's even slightly abnormal will be sensed earlier, felt more intensely, and will linger longer, making it harder to treat.

For example, let's consider how fibromyalgia can complicate the treatment of people who suffer from carpal tunnel syndrome.

It can be all but impossible in such cases to tell how much of the pain can be attributed directly to carpal tunnel complications and how much is simply due to the lowering of the pain threshold.

Figure 9 - Carpal Tunnel Syndrome

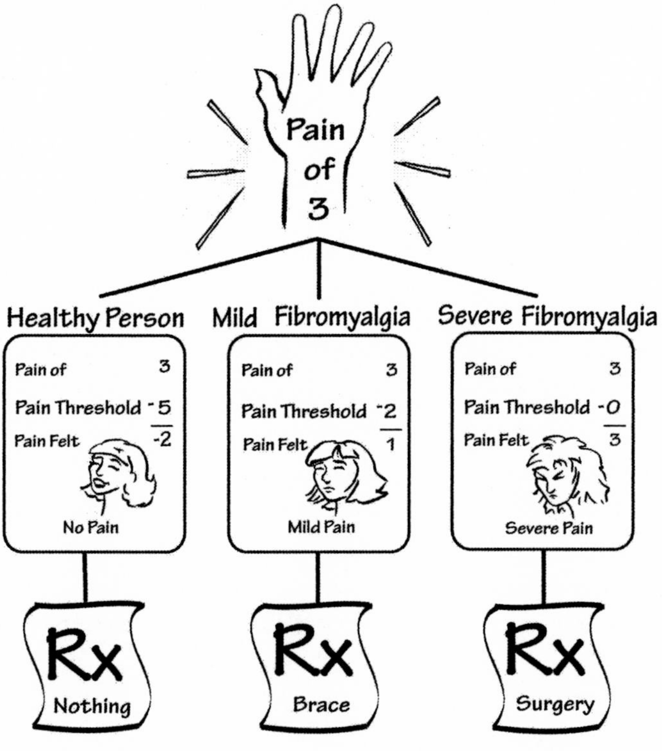

When someone with carpal tunnel syndrome (a painful compression of the nerves of your hand) has a pain of three the degree of pain can range from no pain to severe pain, depending on the pain threshold (Figure 9). Someone with normal dopamine levels and normal pain threshold will feel no pain. Someone with mild fibromyalgia will feel mild pain and use a brace. Someone with severe fibromyalgia and depleted dopamine will probably feel like they need surgery.

Figure 10 - Carpal Tunnel Syndrome

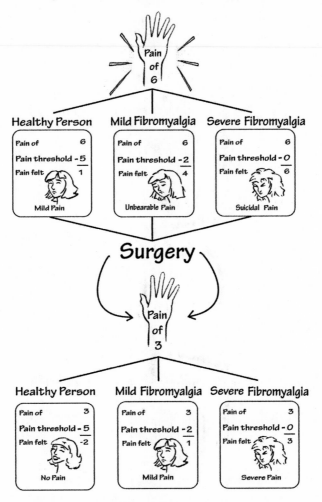

As the carpal tunnel symptoms increase for each person, they all become eligible for surgery (Figure 10). Surgery lessens the amount of painful compression in all three people. With normal levels of dopamine, no pain is felt after surgery. However, with lower levels of dopamine, the normal amount of residual compression following surgery is felt as mild pain. With greatly depleted levels of dopamine, the surgery may appear to have been unsuccessful.

In addition to problems that cause pain, depleted dopamine levels affect every single thing the body is capable of sensing. I once treated a police officer that was unable to sleep because of an intense crawling sensation he experienced all over his body. The sensations were greatly intensified whenever the officer was under stress, particularly if he'd just recently had a lot of difficult interactions with the public or even with his sergeant. He also noticed that the crawling sensations decreased whenever he was away on vacation. He was beginning to think that perhaps he was allergic to his patrol car, his uniform, or perhaps even his house. As he experienced his uncomfortable sensations more at night while he was home, a naturopath had diagnosed him as having multiple chemical sensitivity syndrome and encouraged him to completely redesign his home to eliminate the offending substances. This the officer had done, and yet he was still miserable at night.

Understandably, he become more frustrated and the problem only got worse as a consequence. He endured three more years of being tested by allergists, dermatologists, and neurologists, all to no avail. After all that, the officer's primary care physician was at a total loss as to how to proceed.

That's when he came to me expecting yet another disappointment. I quickly saw that he suffered from stress, depression, and restless legs. What's more, he verified that his crawling sensations varied in step with these fibromyalgia causes. That's why it came as no surprise to me that his symptoms improved whenever he was on vacation whereas they worsened whenever his relations with his sergeant grew tense.

I explained to him that fibromyalgia was the cause of his sensations and that this was a very curable situation. He was dubious at first — not surprising, given all that he'd already been through. I persuaded him to take a medication that would increase his dopamine levels. Even at a very low dosage, he was amazed to find that the crawling disappeared in just under a month.

At this point he understood that his problem related entirely to his adrenaline levels, and he dropped the medication and started working on other techniques for minimizing stress and depression. Eventually, his problem was resolved.

Many health care providers will tell their fibromyalgia patients that their problems are just a matter of nerves or stress. This is partly correct. But unless a person can understand how stress actually causes the amplified sensations that lead to so much pain and distress, it's almost impossible to make progress towards a remedy. The whole purpose of this book is to get people past that hurdle with clear explanations and practical techniques that can be employed by anyone with the core problems that lead to fibromyalgia.

Does heredity play a role?

Many patients insist that fibromyalgia runs in their families. Rest assured, you were not born with fibromyalgia. It is possible, however, that some other genetic predispositions could be at play. Perhaps a previously unknown cause of fibromyalgia runs in the family, such as lupus or bipolar disorder. Similarly, an abusive, alcoholic father could have a major hand in ensuring a life of fibromyalgia struggles for all of his children. Fibromyalgia is not in the genes. Neither is it contagious. But the causes of it, especially stress, anxiety, and depression, can be readily communicated from person to person and from generation to generation.

Although fibromyalgia is not a genetic disease, certain families may be more inclined than others to high adrenaline levels, due to how they interact with one another and lead their lives rather than because of their genetic makeup. If you think fibromyalgia runs in your family, you should probably start to look for those causes the family seems to have in common. The possibilities range from a family predisposition to lupus to sleep apnea, or even domestic violence.

Anything that serves to raise your adrenaline level puts you one step closer to fibromyalgia. So it's important to identify and start working on your causes, not only so your own condition can be remedied but also to better protect your children from the same suffering you've endured. My own sense is that when children grow up in environments capable of engendering PTSD, the brain "learns" to throttle up the adrenaline level at just the slightest provocation. So, viewed in that way, the single best thing to do to shield your children from a future with fibromyalgia is to simply create the healthiest home environment you can.

A child who grows up with anxiety and insults is one that's likely to grow up in a state of increased adrenaline. This is the sort of background I commonly find with many of my fibromyalgia patients. An anxiety-filled upbringing is also one of the most common causes of PTSD.

The first sign that something is amiss may be that the child experiences intense growing pains or does not socialize very well in school. If you notice anything of the sort with your children, you really need to ask yourself if the household environment might be part of the problem. If so, your children may already be on the road to a life of abnormal adrenaline cycling and painfully amplified sensations.

Why do more women than men get fibromyalgia?

Everyone has a fight or flight response and it works fundamentally the same for each of us. Men have a slight genetic advantage because it generally takes an accumulation of more causes to make their adrenaline cycle abnormally. Women, on the other hand, tend to be genetically predisposed to higher adrenaline levels. As a consequence, most of the people who suffer from fibromyalgia are women, and this may also help to explain why some women seem to have more than their fair share of health complaints.

Roughly 90 percent of the patients I see are women. Part of the answer may lie in a study done in London back in the

1970s, in which three physicians — Davis, Nodal and Charnock — at the National Hospital for Nervous Diseases developed a computer-assisted technique for monitoring people's breathing without disturbing them. One of their interests had to do with studying the differences between male and female sleep patterns. They discovered the differences are actually quite striking. This study provides proof that it is much easier to interrupt a woman's sleep than to rouse a man. In my view, this gives us good reason to believe that these same genetic differences may also explain why it is easier to raise a woman's adrenaline level.

Don't curse your genetics. This is likely a very important component of our genetic makeup as women respond to hearing their baby cry at night. Without this genetic difference in sleep, a crying or sick baby would go unattended.

In another study, Shelly Taylor of UCLA found that a woman's fight and flight response works differently than a man's. Specifically, women "tend and befriend" as a response to stress to protect themselves and their offspring. Their brains make different stress chemicals and in different amounts. This is yet another example of the differences observed in men versus women's fight or flight response.[2]

Although women often have more problems with improperly cycling adrenaline, men are not immune to fibromyalgia.

It just takes a few more causes for men to cross the threshold and start manifesting the symptoms of fibromyalgia. This is why it's always a good idea to carefully look for secondary causes such as lupus and sleep apnea whenever men are diagnosed with fibromyalgia. Of course, it's actually a good practice to check for secondary causes in all such cases, regardless of sex, before embarking on fibromyalgia treatments.

Why do so many people with fibromyalgia feel confused?

Confusion is such a familiar symptom of fibromyalgia that it commonly is referred to as "fibro fog." Patients with fibromyalgia frequently have difficulty with memory recall, both short-term and long-term. The fibromyalgia link to confusion has been demonstrated in multiple studies. These studies also indicate that fibromyalgia tends to reduce mental alertness (concentration), diminish test performance, and slow the speed at which people are able to complete complex cognitive tasks.[3]

In another study, Dr. John Newcomer of the University of Washington at St. Louis set out to assess the effect of stress on memory performance. By dosing healthy people with cortisol, one of the hormones released during stress, Dr. Newcomer was able to induce memory and concentration problems similar to those found with fibromyalgia patients.[4]

The relationship between stress and "fibro fog" is actually easy to understand. Most of your sensations and many of your thoughts travel through the limbic system, one of the busiest traffic centers in your brain. When your fight or flight response is on high alert, the brain is constantly analyzing your environment for potential threats. Therefore you're real good at getting startled, angry or upset. It's no wonder your limbic system assigns a low priority to thought processes having to do with recalling where you left your car keys. However, as soon as your adrenaline starts to return to normal, your car keys can be given a bit more attention.

As long as your brain is preoccupied with impending threats to your life, you can expect all other thought processes to be treated as little more than background noise.

What is the connection between lupus and fibromyalgia?
Lupus (an auto-immune disease with widespread pain and many other symptoms) is a common cause of fibromyalgia. I believe it is so common that much of the suffering typically associated with lupus stems directly from fibromyalgia. Lupus sufferers, for example, often have cognitive problems ranging from difficulties with concentration to simple forgetfulness to psychosis and hallucinations. In the instance of seizures, psychosis, or hallucinations, fibromyalgia is surely not to blame.

But when it comes to the simple confusion that so many lupus sufferers report, the subsequent development of fibromyalgia is almost always to blame. I've found with my own lupus patients that their level of confusion tended to increase whenever they were also confronted with other fibromyalgia causes — such as high stress or poor sleep.

HOW CAN I DISTINGUISH BETWEEN FIBROMYALGIA AND OTHER PROBLEMS?

Now that we've looked at how fibromyalgia can amplify every sensation in your body and what the implications of that can be, it's equally important to consider what fibromyalgia is not responsible for. In part, this is so you'll be better able to distinguish between fibromyalgia and any other problems that may be ailing you. At times, I've been aware of patients and health care practitioners alike who just *assumed* that every pain or symptom they observed was due solely to fibromyalgia. The truth is that there are times when far more serious problems might also be at play. Learning how to distinguish between fibromyalgia and those other problems requires extensive experience and training. However, just by reading this book, you'll become much more familiar with fibromyalgia and what can and cannot be attributed to it.

Is it possible to have Chronic Fatigue Syndrome (CFS) and fibromyalgia at the same time?

Although most patients with fibromyalgia suffer from overwhelming fatigue, the probability of you having both CFS and fibromyalgia at the same time is extremely low. The overwhelming fatigue of CFS is caused by a chronic persistent infection often associated with sore throat, fever, and swollen glands. The fatigue associated with fibromyalgia is due to improperly cycling adrenaline. This is why the fatigue from fibromyalgia will vary with the fibromyalgia causes and the fatigue from an infection will not.

In my opinion, most of the people diagnosed with CFS actually don't have a chronic infection. Instead, many are probably suffering from fibromyalgia or depression rather than CFS. People can think for years that they're battling a chronic infection such as the Epstein-Barr Virus or Candida, when in fact they'd be better able to actually *do* something about their fatigue if they had a proper diagnosis. Sometimes in these cases, I've found that the patients weren't initially diagnosed with fibromyalgia simply because they didn't exhibit the classic fibromyalgia tender points. That's why it's so very important to also look for other telltale signs of fibromyalgia.

In the past it was assumed that everything that happens to a person with fibromyalgia was caused by the fibromyalgia.

Although fibromyalgia patients are far more aware of a host of other conditions, fibromyalgia does not cause these conditions. This could include a heightened awareness of allergies, chronic sinus pain, yeast infections, painful fluid retention in the ankles and feet (edema), headaches (including migraines), plantar fasciitis (tendonitis in the arches of your feet) as well as any other instances of tendonitis or bursitis, growing pains, hypoglycemia, endometriosis, painful menses, fibrocystic breast disease, irritable bowel syndrome, depression, frequent colds, morning stiffness, sunburns, muscle twitching, insect bites, ingrown toenails, adverse reactions to medications, dry skin, sore throat, PMS, TMJ syndrome, Lyme disease, dry eyes or mouth. Mind you, none of these things in their own right are pleasant. But, with fibromyalgia, they can become downright unbearable.

A few of these amplified complaints are common enough (or severe enough) that they deserve some attention in their own right:

Irritable Bowel Syndrome (IBS)

IBS can involve abdominal pain, heartburn, constipation, or diarrhea. Besides being a very common problem, IBS is also thought to be linked to many of the same causes that lead to fibromyalgia – including stress, poor sleep, PTSD, depression, and anxiety. But here's an important distinction: your intestines have their own local nervous system, which will react in its own way to increased adrenaline levels. Different chemicals are involved than those in the workings of fibromyalgia. Still, it's quite likely that the bowel learns to behave in an aberrant manner from years of coping with the fight or flight response, in the same way the central nervous system makes the sort of adjustments that can lead to fibromyalgia.

Infections

Fibromyalgia does not cause infections. However, your immune system will not operate at top efficiency with excessive adrenaline levels. What's more, you're certain to feel every infection all that much more intensely whenever your sensations are perceived as amplified. Fevers and chills will feel more intense, muscle aches from the flu may become unbearable, and the urge to cough will increase as any secretions in the throat are felt more intensely.

Even though fibromyalgia can't be blamed for *causing* your infection, it does make a substantial difference all the same – namely, you'll feel the infection sooner, the symptoms will be more intense, the infection may seem to run a longer course, and it will be harder to resolve all the symptoms. As you're probably gathering, fibromyalgia tends to exaggerate the symptoms and to complicate the treatment of just about all ailments.

Depression

Many patients also insist that they'd never felt depressed *until* fibromyalgia became a part of their life. This isn't surprising since, once you've entered the cycle of fibromyalgia, both the situation and the pain can have a depressing effect. As a physiological condition, depression serves to further raise your adrenaline levels since your body makes the same adrenaline with depression as it does in a car accident. This, in turn, contributes to the vicious cycle of fibromyalgia and increases your pain. Being stuck in a cycle of pain and fatigue can make anyone irritable, angry, desperate, despondent, and hopeless. This explains why fibromyalgia can often lead to divorce, lost jobs, and many other personal disasters. Each of these tragedies in turn makes its own contribution to worsening the vicious cycle of fibromyalgia.

It's a mistake to assume that everyone with fibromyalgia is depressed. It's quite common to find people with fibromyalgia who aren't in the least bit depressed. In my own practice, for example, I see far more fibromyalgia patients with Type-A personalities than with depression. This makes perfect sense to me, as people with Type-A personalities are usually highly accomplished and motivated people who basically live in a constant state of stress and high adrenaline. Because their adrenaline baselines are so high to start with, most of these people don't start showing signs of fibromyalgia until they've acquired enough other causes of fibromyalgia to push their adrenaline levels over the top.

Why do some people with fibromyalgia experience skin flushing?
Skin flushing (that is, the sort of red marks that appear whenever you rub your skin vigorously) is one of a number of things that are certainly related to fibromyalgia, but are actually caused by elevated adrenaline levels. Whenever your adrenaline flow is increased (for whatever reason), blood vessels in your arms and legs dilate — increasing the flow of blood into those areas. If you were being chased by a saber-toothed tiger, that added surge of oxygen-rich blood to your extremities might give you just the boost needed to help you make your escape. As it is, the increased blood flow to your extremities probably does little more than redden your skin — and perhaps release some heat (almost literally "let off some steam").

Still, the association between flushing skin and fibromyalgia is close enough that "skin rolling" was once employed as one of the primary diagnostic criteria for fibromyalgia. That is, the person performing the diagnosis would simply roll the patient's skin between their fingers to see if an abnormal red or swollen reaction resulted. We know now, however, that this test actually serves only to detect increased adrenaline levels – something that may signify nothing more than anxiety about the examination itself.

Now that you have a better understanding of what fibromyalgia is actually doing to you, let's start to examine some of the treatment possibilities available.

CASE
STUDY

MARGARET H.

Sixty-year old Margaret went from doctor to doctor trying to find out why she was hurting so badly. She was experiencing a great deal of pain trying to care for the animals on her farm. Here's what she had to say about her experience with Dr. Dryland.

MAJOR SYMPTOMS

"I'm a very busy person. In addition to those animals, I had a whole bunch more responsibilities. I had a big greenhouse where I grew hydroponic vegetables. When I was sick, I couldn't do anything but go to work – that was the extent of my day. The other thing about fibromyalgia is they can't diagnose it. I was sent to doctor after doctor trying to figure out what was going on."

RESULTS

"I would say it was almost 100 percent better. It's great to feel better. But you still have to work on it, like you still have to exercise and get the sleep that you need, but you're able to do it!"

~

CASE
STUDY

GAIL M.

Gail M. felt relieved to finally be listened to by a doctor when she went in and spoke with Dr. Dryland. Here's what she said when he explained the cause and treatment of fibromyalgia.

"To be believed is a great relief. To be told that glands in my body are the culprits mercifully establishes fibromyalgia as a reality. To learn of a medicine that can control the glands is to return my hope and visions of a future. To be assured that I did not cause the terrible stress that imbalanced my glands is to release my guilt and unleash my inner confidence and strength. And, to experience increased energy and diminished pain is to restore my zest and joy of living."

~

CHAPTER 5

What Can I Do About Fibromyalgia?

People with fibromyalgia have four treatment options. Each of these options can be beneficial, but only the last two of these options are capable of making a permanent improvement. These are also the two treatment possibilities that have been largely overlooked. They won't be overlooked here, though, since we'll explore each of these approaches in depth.

1) Take medications for immediate relief.
2) Seek treatments that make your body feel better.
3) Work on the causes to better regulate your adrenaline.
4) Use a medication to regulate your adrenaline.

But first, let's take a closer look at the two more conventional treatment options.

MEDICATIONS FOR IMMEDIATE RELIEF

Providing medications for immediate relief is how the majority of the medical community currently chooses to treat fibromyalgia. Admittedly, the medications do make a difference, which is why I prescribe them myself. However, achieving a bit of immediate relief should never be confused with being cured. The medications in question here are the same ones that are typically prescribed for insomnia, pain, depression, anxiety, tense muscles, or to slow nerve conduction. Let's take a closer look at each type of medication in turn.

Medicating for sleep.

Of all the medications currently prescribed for fibromyalgia sufferers, those that provide for better sleep are certainly among the most important. That's because it's absolutely vital that you get your adrenaline cycling normally again. Just by normalizing your sleep cycle, you stand to make tremendous headway in that regard. This is why more sleep can make such a significant difference in your battle against fibromyalgia, even if you're unable to effectively address any of your other causes.

A lack of sleep is probably one of the most important causes of fibromyalgia.

Some even believe a lack of sleep may be the only cause. It's been my experience that more than just a lack of sleep typically contributes to the chronically high adrenaline levels associated with fibromyalgia.

That's why, with patients who can't otherwise get enough quality sleep, I recommend sleep medications such as over-the-counter Benadryl, or I prescribe medications such as Ativan or Xanax until such time as their adrenaline starts to cycle normally again. As we proceed into efforts to actually affect a cure, patients can usually stop these medications.

Medicating for pain.

Medications for pain include anti-inflammatories, narcotics, and muscle relaxants. Although treating pain is certainly important, it turns out that narcotic pain medications don't work all that well when someone is suffering from a severe case of fibromyalgia. In my experience, I have discovered why narcotics don't work well in fibromyalgia. The main way narcotics inhibit pain is through in-creasing dopamine activity in the limbic system. Since dopamine is depleted in fibromyalgia, it is no wonder that narcotics don't work well. The more severe your fibromyalgia causes, the more dopamine will be depleted and the less effective narcotics will be. The fibromyalgia cycle itself makes narcotics less effective. So, you were a set-up for disappointment before you ever swallowed your first Vicodin.[1] Patients who take narcotics such as Vicodin or Percocet usually get some temporary relief, but it's sure to wear off in short order. It's not long before many of these patients are back looking for more narcotics – and at higher dosages. It also explains why many physicians are reluctant to prescribe narcotic pain medications for patients with fibromyalgia.

Most health care providers who treat fibromyalgia patients with high doses of narcotics can attest that the pain these pa-tients feel never really goes away, and, in addition to the physical pain, many also manage to add the shame and hopelessness of drug addiction. In many ways narcotics can be counterproduc-tive because they rely on the patient's already depleted dopamine levels to provide temporary pain relief. As a result, the patient's dopamine level plummets further still, and so yet another cycle of misery is perpetuated.

In my experience, should you find that narcotics are actually very helpful for you, it's likely you're treating an additional prob-lem – perhaps what you have instead is arthritis or tendonitis. This is why my own practice, I generally prescribe low doses of narcotics adequate to cover a 24-hour period, while almost never allowing that dose to escalate. Instead, I prefer to keep my treat-ments focused on where the real fibromyalgia problem resides, namely on the patient's elevated adrenaline level.

Muscle relaxants, such as Flexeril, can also be helpful for tem-porary pain relief and improved sleep. Neurontin and a related drug called Pregabalin are also useful, since they work to slow nerve conduction, reducing pain and even anxiety.

Medicating for depression & anxiety.

For certain people suffering from fibromyalgia, medications for depression and anxiety can be quite helpful if these are current causes of your fibromyalgia. Fibromyalgia remains misunderstood throughout much of the medical community, and some health care providers tend to give anti-depressant medications to all fibromyalgia patients. Of course, if you don't happen to be depressed, these medications aren't likely to do much to help regulate your adrenaline. Many anxiety medications, on the other hand, can be quite helpful for sleep, but only if restricted to evening use. Whenever possible, I try to get patients who are already taking anxiety medications (including Klonipin, Ativan, Valium, Xanax) to take them only in the evening to better encourage their adrenaline to cycle more normally.

Hormone Replacement Therapy (HRT).

Women take HRT to alleviate the hot flashes, interrupted sleep, and other symptoms of menopause. Because of the recently discovered cancer risks associated with hormone replacement therapy, many fibromyalgia patients have chosen to end their HRT regimens. Observation has shown that many of these patients tend to do worse on the fibromyalgia front once this happens. Thus, if you stop your HRT treatments and find that you're sleeping worse, feel more stressed or notice anything else that might indicate an elevated adrenaline level, you may want to reconsider HRT use. It may be perfectly acceptable for you to take only the most modest dose of HRT required to relieve your symptoms until such time the HRT is no longer needed. Speak to your health care provider to see what approach may be best for you.

TREATMENTS THAT MAKE YOUR BODY FEEL BETTER

Each and every pain or uncomfortable feeling that you associate with fibromyalgia is occurring at some level in your body. The more you can calm down these areas of your body, the less intense those uncomfortable sensations are likely to be when they are perceived as amplified in your brain.

Exercise can be very helpful in this regard unless your fibromyalgia is quite severe. The best advice I can offer here is that you should do what you can, backing off whenever sharp pains indicate that you've gone too far. Also, should a pain wait until the next day to appear – that too should be taken as a sign that you've probably done too much. In terms of treating any muscle pain, heat is usually best, but severe pains or muscle spasms should probably be iced. For example, should you start to hurt more after spending some time in a hot tub, your fibromyalgia is likely at a severe level, meaning you should probably use ice to treat your sore areas until things calm down.

If you are red hot with fibromyalgia and perceive amplified sensations to an extreme extent, even the slightest pulls and aches are likely to feel unbearable. This also explains why massage may be helpful for you some days while it hurts other days. Similar reasoning applies to most of the treatments you might typically seek to make your body feel better, including physical therapy, chiropractic and osteopathic manipulation, acupuncture, bodywork, yoga, reflexology, stretching, acupressure, and craniosacral therapy. Also, for similar reasons, certain pillows or bedding that you might normally favor may cause you problems during your fibromyalgia flare-ups.

Fibromyalgia patients find it truly maddening that what their body can and can't take is apt to change on a daily basis. However, as you monitor your causes and how fluctuations in those are mirrored in your amplified sensations, you'll start to get a much better sense for what you can expect. That is, whenever your causes are muted, your dopamine will build back up and you'll be able to tolerate more that day. Conversely, on days when your causes are particularly bad, you'll know it's best not to do anything that might possibly aggravate the situation as this will further deplete your dopamine stores.

For example, let's say you take a vacation on some tropical resort. Many people with fibromyalgia are likely to feel better towards the end of such a vacation. Also, they're apt to sleep better as their pain becomes less intense. But then, within a few weeks of returning to the daily grind their pain and fatigue return.

The truth about fibromyalgia is that each real problem gets your attention sooner, hurts you more, becomes harder to treat, and lasts longer.

This doesn't suggest for an instant that you should take any of your pains any less seriously. In fact, you probably will need to pay more attention so you can start to learn more about what you can and can't do during the recovery process. This applies to how you participate in sports activities, how you use your workstation, how you play with your kids, how you go about your housework, the sexual practices you engage in, your travel routines, and just about anything else that might put physical stress on your body.

While treatments designed to make your body feel better are entirely viable, they are quite involved. What's more, a long-term commitment is required since the goal is to treat the symptoms of fibromyalgia – not to cure it. However, taking these steps to make your body feel better will give you the strength and energy necessary to work on the causes.

If it's a proactive cure that you're looking for, there are only two options that will raise your dopamine level: 1) Work to reduce or eliminate the causes of fibromyalgia, and/or 2) Use a medication to replace your depleted dopamine stores.

WORK ON THE CAUSES

Going right to work on the problems that cause fibromyalgia is always my preferred treatment option. But, as many of my patients have reminded me, "Easier said than done." One even went so far as to ask, "What if I happen to live on Planet Earth?" Point well taken. Clearly, if someone were somehow able to magically turn off their stress and start sleeping well, chances are they'd be doing it already.

I've also found that people are much more motivated about working on their causes once they're able to see the direct relationship to the painful symptoms they have to endure. It's really just as simple as that; the more you can do to reduce stress and get more sleep, the more your dopamine will build up and the less pain, confusion and fatigue you're likely to experience.

I've already discussed the relationship between the causes of fibromyalgia and the vicious cycle they feed into. I've also explained the direct relationship between variances in the causes and the intensity of the symptoms. But what you may not fully appreciate quite yet is just how strong the link is between causes and symptoms. In addition to the causes that initially triggered your case of fibromyalgia, you now may also have other causes that were themselves created by your fibromyalgia. This is why fibromyalgia hangs on so stubbornly and is so very hard to treat.

For example, let's say that dealing with your fibromyalgia has resulted in depression. As we discussed in Chapter 3, your depression is likely to wreak further havoc on your adrenaline cycling, which in turn will serve to heat up your fibromyalgia. Effect becomes cause. In fact, anything that is currently pushing your adrenaline level higher has to be considered a current cause of your fibromyalgia – even if it had absolutely nothing whatsoever to do with triggering your fibromyalgia in the first place.

In order to make it easier to sort things out, the following material on how to address your causes has been broken down into three general categories:

1) **Sleep**

2) **Psychological**

3) **Pain**

1) Dealing with sleep issues.

Providing for improved sleep is tremendously important for anyone looking to get the upper hand in the battle against fibromyalgia. If you think you sleep well, but awaken tired or know you snore, the first step is to investigate whether you have sleep apnea. If so, treatments should begin as soon as possible. Even subtle cases of sleep apnea can raise your adrenaline level since any reduction in your oxygen levels during your sleep time can result in high-alert adrenaline cycling throughout the whole night.

This is why it's extremely difficult to make headway against fibromyalgia while even a mild case of sleep apnea remains untreated. So if you've already been diagnosed with sleep apnea but have found it difficult to use CPAP (a breathing device designed to help people combat the problem), you should try again. It can take months to get used to wearing a CPAP mask, but it may prove to be well worth the effort. There also are a number of other options for treating sleep apnea, some of which are surgical. If you are still having problems with sleep apnea, I recommend that you talk to your doctor about different treatment options.

Sleep apnea can also lead to weight gain, obesity, high blood pressure and a host of other health problems. While combating fibromyalgia should probably be a strong enough argument in its own right, there also are many other reasons for aggressively treating sleep apnea. But let's say sleep apnea has already been ruled out. What else can you do to encourage better sleep?

Here are a few options:

- Sleep only when sleepy to reduce the amount of time you lie awake in bed.
- If you can't fall asleep within 20 minutes, get up and do something tedious until you feel sleepy. But don't expose yourself to bright light since the light cues to your brain that it's time to wake up. One option may be to simply sit in the dark until you feel yourself nodding off.
- Don't take naps. This is to ensure that you're tired when it's time to go to bed. And if you absolutely can't make it through the day without a nap, make sure you keep it to less than an hour and complete it before 3 p.m.
- Get up and go to bed at the same time each and every day – even on weekends! Once you establish a regular rhythm in your sleep pattern, you'll find it's easier to fall asleep, and you'll also feel better.
- Refrain from exercise at least four hours prior to bedtime. Regular exercise is certainly recommended to help you sleep well, but timing your workouts intelligently is also important. Exercise in the morning or early afternoon should not interfere with your sleep. Also morning exercise will raise your metabolism for the entire day and is likely to help you lose weight.
- Develop sleep rituals. It's important to give your body unmistakable cues that it's time to slow down and sleep. Listen to relaxing music, read something soothing for 15 minutes, have a cup of caffeine-free tea or do some relaxation exercises.
- Use your bed only for sleeping. Refrain from using your bed as a platform for watching television, paying bills, working or reading. What you really want is for your mind to associate your bed with sleeping – so that when you go to bed, your body will know for certain that it's time to sleep.
- Stay away from caffeine, nicotine and alcohol at least 4-6 hours prior to bedtime. Caffeine and nicotine are stimulants

that interfere with your ability to fall asleep. Among the substances to beware of are coffee, cigarettes, tea, cola, cocoa, chocolate and some prescription and non-prescription drugs.

- While it may seem at first that alcohol helps you get to sleep since it slows brain activity, it generally leads to a night of fragmented sleep.

- Have a light snack before bed. If your stomach is too empty when you go to bed, that could end up interfering with your sleep. However, a heavy meal just prior to bedtime is equally likely to interfere. A better bet is a light snack consisting of dairy products and turkey, both of which contain tryptophan, a natural sleep inducer.

- Make sure your bed and bedroom are quiet and comfortable. A hot room can be uncomfortable, so a cooler room supplied with enough blankets to keep you warm is recommended. In the event that light in the early morning bothers you, get a blackout shade or wear a slumber mask.

- If noise bothers you, wear earplugs or make use of a "white noise" machine, such as a fan. Take a hot bath 90 minutes before bedtime. A hot bath will raise your body temperature, of course, but it's the drop in body temperature that follows that may leave you feeling sleepy.

- Use sunlight to set your biological clock As soon as you get up in the morning, go outside and turn your face to the sun for 15 minutes. This helps regulate your sleep/wake cycle.

- I strongly recommend the book, *Say Goodnight to Insomnia,* by Dr. Gregory Jacobs. I consider it required reading for anyone who has trouble sleeping. The book is especially helpful for fibromyalgia sufferers as it explores the link between stress and sleep, offering intelligent treatment tips as it goes.

Finally, jobs that require you to work night shifts – or worse yet, involve varying shifts should be avoided. People need regular and predictable sleep schedules, so it's no surprise that shift work has often been found to worsen fibromyalgia cases. This admonition also applies to patients who travel frequently for work, especially if that involves changing time zones.

Should you feel that maintaining a normal, regular sleep schedule is not feasible given your current situation, you may find that taking melatonin helps to some degree. If all else fails, I recommend talking to your doctor about sleep medications.

2) Dealing with psychological causes.

Psychological issues can be scary and difficult, and yet ultimately satisfying to treat. That's because the payoff for achieving break-throughs on the psychological front can be dramatic. Not only will your pain and fatigue diminish as a consequence, but you'll also probably be happier and able to start enjoying life again – which in turn should help to start your adrenaline cycling more normally. And, make no mistake, depression among fibromyalgia sufferers is extremely common. It's easy to get depressed when you're tired, wracked with pain and see no way out. That's why it's so important to never lose sight of the fact that fibromyalgia sufferers stand to realize tremendous improvements whenever their causes are appropriately treated. Fibromyalgia is not neces-sarily the life sentence it may seem to be.

So let's quickly review the psychological causes that often play a role in fibromyalgia: stress, depression, generalized anxiety and/or panic disorders, PTSD, bipolar disorder, and schizophre-nia, among others. The main thing each of these has in common is that they all end up raising your adrenaline level.

In general, you have four options available to you for treating the psychological causes of fibromyalgia. Any of these choices can be implemented in any combination you choose:

a) Self help.

There are many excellent self-help books that can help with anxiety, depression and sleep issues. In addition to self-help books, the other self-help options for those looking to deal with their psychological causes are biofeedback, hypnosis (either self-induced or attained with the assistance of a professional hypnotist), meditation and other personal growth work. Basically, feel free to explore any method that you feel may prove effective in reducing your adrenaline level.

b) Therapy.

A qualified therapy professional can help you identify the psychological causes that are most at play in your fibromyalgia, and can introduce you to strategies for better managing those issues. To identify the best therapist for you, referrals from friends and loved ones can be useful, but you may also want to consult with your primary health care provider to identify professionals with a proven expertise in treating your particular causes. In addition to traditional counseling, there are other forms of therapy you might explore. In the end, all that matters is that the program you choose is the one that works best to lower your adrenaline level, reduce your fatigue, and turn down the perceived amplification of your sensations.

c) Medications.

In addition to self-help and therapy, prescription medications may be necessary. For some, including people with schizophrenia, there really is no other option. This can also be true for those with bipolar disorder. Even in cases of depression and anxiety, many people find that these medications can help to break the vicious cycle of fibromyalgia.

d) Take control of your fight or flight response.

Learning to properly use fight or flight response is critical to curing not only fibromyalgia, but all forms of stress, anxiety, fear, and depression. The fight or flight response is the focus of my work. My seminars and upcoming book, *Taking Control of Your Fight or Flight Response: An Instruction Manual for the Human Brain*, can help you use your own fight or flight response to your advantage. You'll find more information on this in Chapter 7.

3) Dealing with pain.

Anything that causes pain will result in higher adrenaline levels. The more intense and prolonged that pain is, the more likely it is to either trigger or worsen your vicious cycle of fibromyalgia. This is why lupus or a car accident can lead to fibromyalgia – which in turn, of course, will only cause anything that's already painful to hurt all the more. So, given this complex interrelationship between pain and fibromyalgia, I'd say you'd be wise to treat any other painful disorder for two fundamental reasons:

- The lower your pain is in the first place, the less agony it's likely to cause once the sensation is perceived as amplified in your brain.
- The fewer pain signals you have to process, the less apt you are to raise your adrenaline level.

It can be difficult sometimes to sort out the aches and pains that result from fibromyalgia from all your other problems. One general rule-of-thumb is that a flu-like, overall achy feeling might well be due to fibromyalgia, while pains that are localized to certain areas are more likely to be due to more specific problems, such as arthritis or tendonitis.

Whenever overwhelming fatigue or confusion accompanies your pains, it's usually reasonable to assume the pains are the result of fibromyalgia.

As always, you should monitor to see whether the pain level varies as changes in other fibromyalgia causes occur. If increased stress equals increased pain, then fibromyalgia is the likely culprit. A good rheumatologist can be particularly helpful in working with you to identify which pains are likely associated with fibromyalgia and which ones aren't.

Even if it turns out that you're unable to treat some of your painful conditions, such as severe osteoarthritis, there still is hope. That's because even if one cause is untreatable, you still have a good chance of netting overall improvement by treating your other causes.

REGULATE YOUR ADRENALINE THROUGH MEDICATION

A new medication approach based on a revolutionary off-label protocol has been shown to be of tremendous value to many fibromyalgia sufferers, with significant improvements noted for virtually everyone who's been able to take the medication. The main problem is that not everyone's body is able to tolerate this regimen of drugs.

This regimen takes advantage of drugs typically used to treat Parkinson's disease. I refer to it as an "off-label protocol" because I'm using it to treat a problem other than the one that is specified "on label" by the Food and Drug Administration (FDA). The drugs included in the protocol are called dopamine agonists, i.e. work like dopamine in your body. These drugs, Mirapex (pramipexole) and Requip (ropinarole), are FDA-approved for the treatment of Parkinson's disease.

It's interesting that drugs developed for the treatment of Parkinson's disease should also be effective in treating fibromyalgia because the two problems are actually nothing at all alike. In contrast to the overactive adrenaline cycling that's characteristic of fibromyalgia, Parkinson's disease has a degenerative effect on the part of the brain that's responsible for producing dopamine, slowing it to a crawl. As a consequence, patients with Parkinson's tend to walk slowly (usually with shuffling steps), move rigidly, write small, stare vacantly, display little facial movement, and often exhibit a resting tremor. And all of this is because of a critical shortage of dopamine. Not surprisingly, treatment largely involves efforts to replenish dopamine levels. Mirapex and Requip work towards this end with agents that bind to just a single dopamine receptor. It's precisely because these drugs are so specific to this single receptor site that both can be administered at higher doses – with fewer side effects.

In 2000, Dr. Andrew Holman published a landmark study showing that it's possible to treat severe fibromyalgia with high doses of these Parkinson's medications.[2] However, it remained unknown exactly how these medications worked until the recent studies performed on laboratory rats demonstrated that replacing dopamine in stressed rats decreased the amount of fibromyalgia pain. I discussed what the data from those studies revealed in Chapter 2.

Dr. Holman's study was the first to demonstrate that replacing dopamine in particular can be an extremely effective way to treat fibromyalgia in humans.

In fact, Mirapex and Requip are both nearly 100 percent effective in treating fibromyalgia. The primary drawback is that only about 50 to 60 percent of patients are currently able to tolerate the medications' side effects over a long period of time. Still, there are many tricks we already know for effectively dealing with these tolerance problems and, with time, it's likely we'll learn even more. As a consequence, I suspect that someday perhaps 75 percent of the people with severe cases of fibromyalgia will be good candidates for Mirapex or Requip treatment programs. As drug development continues, I expect we'll have new dopamine agonists available to us that are much easier to tolerate. The main side effect for fibromyalgia patients – nausea – is also a problem for people who take these medications for Parkinson's disease. So you can rest assured that the pharmaceutical industry is likely working to develop other dopamine agonists that people will find easier to stomach.

I first began using Mirapex with a few of my fibromyalgia patients after meeting with Dr. Holman at a conference in 2001. Dr. Holman is the acknowledged pioneer in the field of dopamine agonists and fibromyalgia. Even though most rheumatologists at the time were highly dubious of Dr. Holman's therapies, the patients I treated with Mirapex soon started to show dramatic improvements. They started thinking clearer and sleeping better. Their energy levels improved and their painful sensations started to resolve. In short, they started to feel as though they'd gotten their lives back.

Needless to say, with these encouraging results, I started using Mirapex with even more of my patients, which is when I learned that only about 50-60 percent of the people I treated could tolerate the side effects. Virtually all of those who were able to take the medication got significantly better. Word spread fast and I soon found more and more fibromyalgia sufferers at my door. Before long, I realized I should report what I'd learned so that other physicians could also make the Mirapex treatment available to their patients. In 2002, I submitted a study to the ACR (the American College of Rheumatology) in which I summarized the results I'd been able to obtain with the first 85 of my patients treated with Mirapex.

Of those 85 patients, 62 were able to take Mirapex – albeit not always at the optimal dose, 4.5 mg. In fact, the average dose people in that initial group were able to handle was 1.9 mg. Of the 62 who were able to take the medication, 58 improved. Each one of these showed at least a 50 percent reduction in his or her pain score over the period covered by the study. Of the 23 patients who were unable to tolerate the medication, nausea was the chief problem reported. A few patients stopped taking the medication due to anxiety, poor sleep, confusion, or bad dreams. Most of the people who stopped taking the medication did so within the first week.

For most people, the pattern of recovery goes like so: first, you'll notice that your body's restless jerking will start to subside. Then you'll find that your sleep improves and your energy grows. After that, you can expect your confusion to clear up. And then, once you're up to the higher doses, you'll find that your sensations aren't quite so amplified anymore and that your pain has subsided. In fact, the improvements that can be realized with Mirapex and Requip are so palpable that even those patients who can't tolerate the drugs well nevertheless opt to stay on a low dose of the medication to gain some partial relief from the miseries of fibromyalgia.

Each of the patients in my practice who benefited was someone who had suffered from a severe case of fibromyalgia.

The dramatic improvements they realized with the medication had an equally dramatic effect on their lives.

They found it hard to believe that a medication capable of making such a dramatic difference in the treatment of fibromyalgia had been available in the pharmacy all along. Now that I have tried Mirapex with over a thousand patients, I have a much better idea of how to administer it, as well as a better sense for the candidates most likely to tolerate it. I've also started to use Requip, the other dopamine agonist therapy that's currently available (Requip, like Mirapex, is also supported by studies published by Dr. Holman). In fact, over the past few years I've even made combined use of Mirapex and Requip with certain patients – with results that have been quite encouraging.

In the paragraphs that follow, I'll try to summarize what I've learned from my experience, so that both you and your primary care physician will have a better idea of what to expect. It's been my experience that many patients who take either Mirapex or Requip might initially suffer with nausea, only to get past all such problems a few weeks later – by which time they're also in significantly less pain than they had been before starting the regimen. Knowing this, I've spent countless hours on the phone encouraging patients not to give up in the early stages. The first thing you need to understand is that the use of Mirapex and Requip discussed here is off-label. That means these drugs have been studied by the manufacturers and evaluated by the Food and Drug Administration for their use in treating Parkinson's disease. These drugs have not been approved for the treatment of fibromyalgia. They also have not been approved for the treatment of the restless legs syndrome.

But does this really matter? Yes, for two reasons. One is that insurance companies may use the fact this is an off-label therapy as an excuse not to pay for expensive drugs. So unfortunately, should you decide to follow this experimental protocol, you may have to pay for it out of your own pocket. It's not unusual for a fibromyalgia sufferer to spend tens of thousands of dollars a year getting tests, seeing different specialists, undergoing surgery for pain relief and obtaining expensive pain-relief medications. The real shame is that very little of this ever works. By contrast, once a patient is on Mirapex and learns to properly use their fight or flight response, their fibromyalgia is usually cured. This certainly will save the insurance industry countless dollars. Dr. Holman is currently engaged in another study designed to demonstrate just how much insurance companies stand to save by encouraging the use of dopamine agonists for the treatment of fibromyalgia patients.

The second implication of using an off-label therapy is much more significant. This is because physicians are required to use special consent forms when they use off-label drugs to guard themselves against potential lawsuits. In a society as litigious as ours, health care providers can be quite reluctant to get involved with off-label therapies. That's understandable, but unfortunately it's the patients who suffer as a result. A model consent form has been included at the end of the *Appendix for Healthcare Providers*.

You may need to use it – or one like it – to alleviate any fear your primary care physician may have in prescribing the dopamine agonists.

In my experience, both drugs are reasonably safe if used very carefully. Neither injures the body in any way. No damaging effects have been observed in the liver, kidney, or any other organ tissues. The only real risk is that people who take these medications can grow sleepy or confused, so caution must always be exercised when driving. You should know that in the *Physician's Desk Reference* there have been reports of auto accidents associated with patients who are using either Mirapex or Requip to treat Parkinson's disease. The key difference to bear in mind is that Parkinson's patients are advised to take the medication around the clock, whereas for fibromyalgia patients the medication should only be used just before bedtime. Also, fibromyalgia patients tend to be much younger than Parkinson's patients, making for an entirely different side-effects profile.

In my own medical practice, I've only had to stop the medication for three patients due to daytime sleepiness (less than one percent of the total number of people who were prescribed either Mirapex or Requip). I also caution each of my patients not to drive if sleepy. Warnings are also included in the consent form I use, and reminders are given at each and every visit.

Beyond sleepiness, the side effects of dopamine agonists can certainly be annoying, but not dangerous to the body in any way. Most patients experience some nausea – roughly 80 percent. In most cases, this is mild and can be treated. Often, the nausea simply goes away with time. Other less likely side effects include anxiety, tremors, worsening sleep, exceptionally vivid dreams, confusion, hallucinations, light-headedness, hair loss, excitation, fluid retention, and tremulousness. But let me emphasize again that these side effects are rare. In my own practice, the only patients I've known to hallucinate on Mirapex are those who also suffer from bipolar disorder.

One troubling side effect is that for people with bipolar disease, Mirapex seems to exacerbate the mania. In a way, this makes sense, as dopamine is essentially a stimulant. When a person becomes unusually talkative or starts to exhibit far too much energy, it may indicate the onset of a manic episode. I even had one patient who started to gamble excessively. When treating bipolar patients, I only prescribe Mirapex according to a program developed in conjunction with the person's psychiatrist, and even then only if provisions have been made for closely monitoring the patient.

I've learned that the people least likely to tolerate these medications are those who already have a history of stomach problems and have already had to stop taking other medications due to stomach problems or nausea. Also, if you are more than 60 years of age, suffer from sleep apnea, or have certain forms of neck arthritis, chances are you may have difficulties with these medications.

There are cases, such as when a patient has sleep apnea, where the advantages afforded by the dopamine agonists may be minimal. If your body thinks it's dying every night (owing to suffocation from sleep apnea), there isn't any drug strong enough to control the corresponding stress response that you get night after night. The significance of this was brought home to me when several patients of mine who didn't respond favorably to Mirapex were eventually found to have sleep apnea.

In addition, certain forms of neck arthritis can raise your adrenaline level – thus undercutting the benefits of Mirapex therapy in much the same way that sleep apnea does. In the 1990s, a specific surgical procedure to relieve this pressure at the base of the brain was one of the more drastic treatments ever tried for fibromyalgia. This procedure can still provide some benefit today whenever neck arthritis is found to be actively contributing to the fibromyalgia cycle.

Taking all of this into account, approximately 20 percent of my patients have had no problem at all with the medication. And for those who can tolerate the dopamine agonists, the encouraging news is that you're almost assured of getting better. Virtually everyone who's able to tolerate a dose over 3 mg of Mirapex is sure to improve, and for many patients, important gains can be realized at even lower doses. For those who've labored with fibromyalgia-induced confusion, the good news is that the confusion is likely to diminish with the use of Mirapex.

So far, this discussion has primarily focused more on Mirapex than on Requip, the other dopamine agonist labeled specifically for Parkinson's treatments. In general, Mirapex is the more effective drug for treating fibromyalgia. However Requip is easier to tolerate and plays a larger role for those patients who have difficulties with Mirapex. I've also found that many patients can tolerate a combination of the two drugs. The side effects for Requip are similar to those for Mirapex, albeit generally not quite so intense. Requip also has one other disadvantage in that it interacts negatively with certain other medications. This gives your health care provider another consideration to account for when developing a medication regimen that's right for you.

Your primary health care provider must be involved in developing this regimen every step of the way. Among other things, that means your physician should be fully familiar with the use of these medications, their implications and potential side effects. That way, should you ever have any concerns you'll know exactly where to turn. Although I have treated over a thousand patients, I'm sure that I have not yet come across every possible side-effect of these medications. This is certainly uncharted territory and there may be some risk with any off-label use of a medication. Use caution, and make sure your physician is aware of any side effects or changes in your body.

In four years of prescribing these medications, I have run across a number of special situations. I've listed some of these below, along with some thoughts on how to interpret and respond to each.

It's possible that you might follow the off-label protocol and yet realize little, if any, progress. In that event, consider the possibility that your pain may be due to something else, such as lupus or osteoarthritis. The dopamine agonists will only provide relief if it's fibromyalgia you're suffering from. Keep in mind that the dopamine agonists are so uniformly effective in the fight against fibromyalgia that you can be reasonably certain that something else is wrong if neither Mirapex nor Requip reduce your discomfort.

Another thing to be aware of is that sleep can at first worsen for some people once they've started to take Mirapex. In those instances – if I feel I can trust the patient not to drive – I have them take their medication in the morning. Then, over time – as the dose gets raised and the patient becomes sleepy from using Mirapex during the day – I ask them to shift over to the more common practice of taking their medication just before bedtime.

For some people, the restless jerking can also worsen before it gets better. In most cases, this will normalize over time. But there are rare instances where it just continues to get worse and worse. In those cases, the medication will have to be stopped. This phenomenon is known as "amplification" and is well known among physicians who regularly treat the restless legs syndrome. Occasionally, the amplification can be overcome with the help of drugs such as Ativan, Xanax, and Klonipin, which are the same drugs I use to lower a patient's adrenaline level enough so they can sleep at night. I also often use these same medications in combination with Mirapex and/or Requip.

Fortunately, Mirapex can be combined with most other medications. In addition, you may be surprised to find that once your adrenaline level has normalized, all of your other medications start to work better. That's particularly true for those medications intended to help you relax or sleep. The same drugs that failed to help you sleep at one time may suddenly become much too strong for you once you've started to replace your dopamine stores. You and your primary health care provider may want to decrease or stop some other medications. For example, it may be that you slipped into a depression over time due to all the pain you were in. But now that your pain has greatly diminished, you may find you no longer need an anti-depressant. The same goes for any pain or sleep medications you may be taking.

Once I start to get better, how much longer should I continue to take these medications?

Either for six months or for a lifetime. If the causes that led to your case of fibromyalgia are truly behind you, as in the case of a car accident, the vicious cycle of fibromyalgia can probably be broken with a few months of Mirapex treatment. But if the causes are still present – whether in the form of lupus, an abusive relationship, Post Traumatic Stress Disorder (PTSD), or depression, you'll probably find that your fibromyalgia will reassert itself within a few weeks or months of stopping the medications.

It is rare for patients to find relief without Mirapex unless they also learn to properly use their fight or flight response.

As for how long it takes to break the fibromyalgia cycle, I've had some patients who could only tolerate a few weeks of Mirapex treatment but still managed to improve to the point where they felt better than they had in years. In each of these cases, the patients were chiefly dealing with the aftermath of the causes initially responsible for trapping them in the vicious cycle of fibromyalgia years earlier.

For all its potential value, some patients also tend to use Mirapex as a crutch. That's why, despite all that Mirapex can do to help alleviate the fibromyalgia symptoms, it is almost never my first option. Whenever it's possible for patients to work on their causes without the help of the off-label protocol, I encourage them to do so. This means that in most of the instances where I do end up prescribing Mirapex, it's only because the pain is so severe it interrupts my efforts to help patients properly learn to use their fight or flight response.

As more and more people start to take the dopamine agonists treatments for fibromyalgia, we'll get a truer, more complete picture of the side effects. My own feeling is that formal studies should already be under way, but unfortunately mine is not the prevailing attitude throughout the medical community. It's largely because of this that I decided to discuss dopamine agonist treatments as part of this book. Dr. Holman is currently working on a book and funding his own small-scale, placebo-controlled trial, but that's no substitute for a larger formal study. Hopefully, it won't be long before one is in the works.

Failing that, I expect the use of Mirapex for the treatment of fibromyalgia to remain off-label for quite some time. One important reason is that Mirapex is so hard to tolerate, and this can make it quite difficult to gain approval for a particular drug application. But, on the other hand, it's also very unusual for a drug to be nearly 100 percent effective. This, of course, is why I've never had reservations about trying Mirapex treatments with my most severe patients. Hopefully, over time, other dopamine agonists will become available that are more readily tolerated. Until then, Mirapex and/or Requip should make a dramatic difference for the patients who are able to tolerate these medications.

The Importance of
True Understanding

"I have seen other doctors. They all looked at me like I was crazy when I talked to them about having been in pain all my life. I've had it my whole life – it started when I was a kid. It goes clear back to my earliest memories. When I went to Dr. Dryland, first and foremost, he didn't look at me like I was crazy. I thought, finally, I've got somebody who had some idea about what I'm going through in life."

– Fred L., Patient

"I had been psychoanalyzed; the psychiatrist basically said that I was faking it. It really upset me because I went through all of these tests because I knew something was wrong. After Dr. Dryland explained to me where fibromyalgia comes from and how the cause can bring on the effects I understood, and agreed that I probably do have fibromyalgia."

– Jude S., Registered Nurse and Patient

"What I really liked about him is that he was thorough, and he took the time to listen to what I had to say. It wasn't like I was just a number in part of a program. I was really a unique individual whom he addressed – that made a tremendous difference."

– Ali D., Patient

"I think he's fantastic. He has a real positive outlook. Whereas most doctors don't even want to test you with fibro, and some of them don't even believe in you he does. He's trying to find help – I really appreciate him."

– Marta S., Patient

"Immediately I knew that I had somebody who understood, and if anything was going to be done for me it was through him. I've been extremely impressed with him."

– Diana F., Registered Nurse and Patient

CHAPTER 6

Explaining Fibromyalgia

Having read most of this book, you now have a much better idea of what fibromyalgia is, how it can affect you, and what you can do about it. Even armed with your new knowledge, it can still be a challenge to explain this diagnosis to the rest of the world. Although many people have heard the word "fibromyalgia", and often nod their heads to indicate understanding when they hear it again, they would be hard-pressed to describe the condition. Also, because there is no visible bodily damage, others may question whether you're truly suffering. They may think you're faking, or that you're simply imagining aches and pains that don't really exist. Often, I've witnessed the added anguish caused by the doubts raised by loved ones and friends. It is important to remember that people can be made uncomfortable by things they do not understand.

Since fibromyalgia has been misdiagnosed and misunderstood for so many years, your challenge is to clearly explain what it really means to have fibromyalgia. In doing so, you will provide your friends, loved ones, and healthcare provider with the tools they need to help you work toward a cure. Sharing information about your condition can be empowering for everyone involved. This chapter will provide you with some ideas for how to explain fibromyalgia to your friends, family, coworkers, and many others.

You can explain fibromyalgia through science-based explanations, physical demonstrations, and by sharing your thoughts and feelings. Your personality, or the personalities of those around you will determine which approach to choose.

Explaining fibromyalgia through science.
The primary reason why fibromyalgia is so misunderstood is because people do not understand the science behind it. I've found that once I provide people with the physiological explanation of how fibromyalgia works, they suddenly become much more interested and empathetic. Here are some suggestions that you can use to explain fibromyalgia:

- Fibromyalgia is not a disease – but it is a very painful and chronic condition that people can develop in association with large amounts of psychological or physical stress.
- The brain cannot tell the difference between physical pain and emotional pain. In either situation, the brain activates the fight or flight response and raises your adrenaline levels. Increased adrenaline levels allow you to run faster, fight harder, and focus more clearly on the situation at hand.
- Dopamine, a type of adrenaline, plays an important role in the fight or flight response. Dopamine effectively blocks the painful sensations that might otherwise keep you from running to safety on an injured leg.
- In situations where chronic physical or emotional stress is ongoing, the body continues to respond with increasing adrenaline. Additionally, if the person is not able to get restful and refreshing sleep, the body will not properly refresh its dopamine stores.
- Fibromyalgia results from this chronic usage of the pain-blocking substance dopamine. As dopamine levels become depleted, a person's normal sensation threshold is greatly reduced. Everyday sensations, as well as painful conditions, are perceived as greatly amplified.

- Fibromyalgia is curable, and does not actually damage the body while it is occurring. However, pain generated from the nervous system can be much more painful than a disfiguring arthritis.
- Depending on who you are talking to, you may want to add your own examples and explain the causes that are unique to your case of fibromyalgia.

Explaining fibromyalgia through physical demonstrations.

One useful way to explain fibromyalgia is to show your friends and family how to identify their own fibromyalgia tender points (See Chapter 2, Figure 2). As described in Chapter 2, these are naturally sensitive areas where pain and any other sensations are greatly amplified once the fibromyalgia cycle is triggered. Ask your friends and loved ones to apply pressure to their own tender points. Is the pressure uncomfortable? Can they tell that we all have a lot of sensitive areas in our bodies? If so, you can explain that you live with these sensations, greatly amplified, all over your body ... every second of every day.

Fibromyalgia patients perceive a wide range of amplified sensations. Ask your friends to remember the last time that they were in a dimly lit or otherwise darkened room for a while, when suddenly the whole room was lit with the bright flash of a camera. Can they remember how everyone moaned and shielded their eyes from the offending flash? The sensitivity that their unprepared eyes experienced during that brief moment is similar to the sensitivity continually experienced by fibromyalgia patients. If they want to know what it's like to experience other amplified sensations, ask them to wear an item of clothing that continually irritates their skin. It could be an irritating seam, a misplaced tag, or the mere texture of the clothing – each of these irritations is probably enough to keep them from wearing that piece of clothing very often. Explain that all of your sensations are heightened in a similar way all the time.

I often tell my patients and their spouses to imagine that they've just worked all day to clean out the garage. Both are sure to have minor muscle aches and strains by the end of the day. But the person with normal dopamine levels will feel these minor problems only slightly – and only when they happen to move in a certain way over the next couple of days. The fibromyalgia sufferer, on the other hand, may end up incapacitated – restricted to a recliner and covered with ice packs for the next week or so. Both likely have the exact same pulled muscle – the only difference being that the person with fibromyalgia has to deal with a greatly amplified pain signal (Figure 11).

Figure 11 - Pain of Six

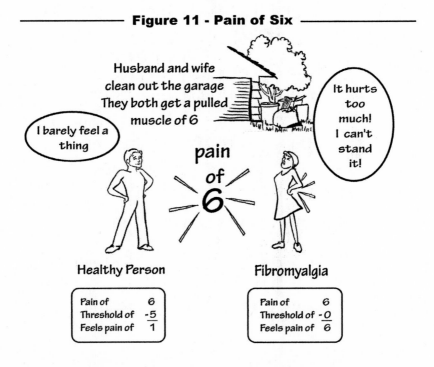

In fact, every sensation can pack a similar wallop. It doesn't really matter whether it's due to cleaning out the garage, undergoing back surgery, suffering a bad case of the flu, or even just getting out of bed in the morning. Each and every sensation can be perceived as amplified to the point where you become thoroughly exhausted and overwhelmed. Fatigue and confusion almost inevitably follow.

Many patients tell me it's almost like having a flu that never ends. Often, it's even much worse — akin, some say, to getting hit by a Mack truck.

Explaining fibromyalgia by sharing thoughts and feelings.
In relationships where you have already developed an emotional connection, one of the easiest ways to explain fibromyalgia is to share your thoughts, feelings, and experiences. Ask your loved ones to think back to the last time they had the flu. Did they feel like having sex? How much interest did they have in going out to the movies? Was it easy to get up in the morning to see the kids off to school? Chances are, they just stayed in bed as much as they could, with only the occasional outing to the bathroom or kitchen. It might have been days before they even thought of leaving the house. Ask them if they can imagine functioning on a day-to-day basis with those symptoms. Explain to them that you don't have the luxury to take those days off because sometimes everyday feels like one of those days.

FIBROMYALGIA AND WORK
In addition to your friends and loved ones, you may also want to explain your fibromyalgia to your employer. Fibromyalgia can dramatically affect a person's ability to be productive at work. If your employer or direct supervisor understands your condition, they may be able to help you create less stressful working conditions with the mutual goal of once again having a highly productive employee. Prior to talking with your employer, make a list of all of the ways that you are still productive in your job. Make

a secondary list of reasonable accommodations that would allow you to be more productive in your current job. These could include:

- Allowing a self-paced workload and flexible hours.
- Allowing you to work from home.
- Providing a part-time work schedule.
- Creating an ergonomically correct workspace.
- Allowing time for medical appointments.

In addition to improving your performance, your employer may also be eligible for tax deductions or business credits, depending on the type of accommodation. If your employer is covered by the employment provisions of the Americans with Disabilities Act (ADA), they are prohibited from discriminating against qualified individuals with disabilities. The following resources can provide you with more information on these topics:

ADA Information Center: 800 949-4232
Job Accommodation Network: 800 526-7234

When talking with your employer, the most important goal to work toward is the creation of a work environment that will benefit both of you.

However, if your goal is to obtain disability compensation, you may be in for some rough sledding. In 1999, the US Social Security Administration included fibromyalgia in its list of disabling conditions. However, this does not mean that everyone with fibromyalgia will be determined to be "disabled." That's because the health care provider relies chiefly on the patient's symptoms to make a diagnosis of fibromyalgia. However, insurance companies and disability review boards would rather see objective data — namely, findings from physical exams, lab reports, radiological scans, surgical reports, or any other measurable findings.

Let's imagine that you developed fibromyalgia in part because of all the stress you endure as an air traffic controller. First of all, where's the hard data to support your claim of fibromyalgia? Secondly, how can you prove that stress from your work environment helped to bring it on? And finally, how can you convince a skeptical supervisor that your current condition interferes with your ability to perform your job? Chances are that people are going to doubt and question your story. In part, that's because people are uncomfortable and rather unforgiving when it comes to any condition that may have a mental or psychological dimension. In our society, the mere mention of anxiety or depression can often be viewed as a sign of weakness.

Nonetheless, there are people who manage to get disability compensation for cases of low back pain, depression, or repetitive strain injuries. All of these lack hard objective evidence. Fibromyalgia should be no different. That is, if the causes of fibromyalgia can be proven, that really should suffice to convince any trained professional of the legitimacy of a fibromyalgia claim.

This may be changing as more and more research confirms my findings regarding fibromyalgia. For example, there now is indisputable scientific evidence that chronic stress or interrupted sleep will lead to amplified pain sensations.[1] Over time, it's likely that much of the rest of my diagnostic criteria will also come to be more commonly accepted and recognized. And that should make the evaluation of fibromyalgia much more straightforward for everyone – including the disability review boards.

As you take inventory of your own life, whichever fibromyalgia causes you find present are almost certainly the culprits responsible for your case of fibromyalgia. The better that you understand your own case of fibromyalgia, the more likely it is that you will be able to explain it clearly to the world around you. Unfortunately, even as you come to grips with fibromyalgia, its underpinnings, and its implications, it still may be difficult to convince some of the people around you of what's happening to you. Sadly, this could include your primary health care provider, who may actually know very little about fibromyalgia or, more likely, be relying on outdated thinking.

Throughout the medical community, there still remains a broad divergence of beliefs regarding what fibromyalgia is actually all about. Some physicians discount its existence altogether. Others care for their fibromyalgia patients appropriately, but are still waiting for better treatments. Others simply ascribe their patients' problems to nothing more than depression. Many patients tell me that most of the people in their lives simply scoff at the idea of fibromyalgia. Some people have even come to believe that fibromyalgia is nothing more than the diagnosis that physicians trot out whenever they have no idea what's going on with a patient. In the past, there may have actually been some truth to that. I'm hoping my diagnostic criteria will help to demystify fibromyalgia, for patients and medical practitioners alike. You may want to show your doctor this book – particularly the *Appendix for Healthcare Providers*.

CASE STUDY

ALI D.

Fifty-two year old Ali D. had a major life breakthrough after working with Dr. Dryland. Here's what she had to say about her experience.

MAJOR SYMPTOMS

"I had an extraordinary experience with Dr. Dryland. I was bedridden because I was in such pain, and then when I did walk I was on crutches. It was probably the darkest point in my life. My diagnosis was fibromyalgia. I'm a fighter, but I was at the point where I didn't know if I wanted to get back up and fight."

RESULTS

"Dr. Dryland talked to me about the off-label protocol and the new things he was trying. He explained to me how it would work. I said okay, because at that point there was no place to go but up. I had an interesting side-effect happen. A friend of mine was kind enough to download to my computer a program where I could open up a canvas and paint. I spent six very intense weeks doing that. I was kind of amazed because I've never been to art school. I produced 30 pieces of work. I did my art to the point that I'm going to have a show in New York sometime this year. That's my incredible story! I find Dr. Dryland to be a doctor of incredible integrity with a genuine concern for his patients. As far as I'm concerned he helped to change my life – completely turn it around!"

~

CHAPTER 7

Moving Beyond Fibromyalgia: Your Plan For a Cure

The best way to treat fibromyalgia is to lower the adrenaline level in your body, thus allowing your limbic system to rebuild its supply of dopamine and start inhibiting sensations once again in a normal fashion. The question is: What's the best way for you to get back to normal adrenaline cycling?

Throughout this chapter, we'll work together to create a personalized plan you can follow to get your life back. There are many other options available to you for achieving some degree of relief – many of which are covered in some of the other books already available on the topic of fibromyalgia. But this book isn't just about relieving the pain of fibromyalgia, it's also about curing fibromyalgia.

The challenge now is to pick the right path for you. Study the following list of fibromyalgia causes. Circle those causes that apply to you. Write down any other causes you may have that are not on this list:

Poor, interrupted or non-refreshing sleep

Sleep apnea

Stress

Anxiety and panic disorders

Depression

Post-Traumatic Stress Disorder

Bipolar disorder/manic-depression

Schizophrenia or other serious psychiatric disorder

Severe osteoarthritis (wear and tear), lupus, rheumatoid arthritis, ankylosing spondylitis, or other painful inflammatory diseases

Painful trauma stemming from an incident, such as a motor vehicle accident

Restless legs syndrome

Hypermobility/double-jointed

As you develop your list, try to probe a bit deeper. For example, if stress is one of your causes, ask yourself: What is it that makes me feel so much stress? What could I change in my life to reduce my stress level? Why is it that I don't sleep very well? When do I seem to have the most difficulty sleeping?

Now, study the following list of symptoms. Again, circle those that are familiar and add more if necessary:

Pain, aching, stiffness, etc.

Numbness, tingling

Itching

Feeling either too hot or too cold

Altered or intensified tastes and smells

Intolerance to bright lights or loud noises

Skin flushing

Uncomfortable being in crowds

Fatigue

Confusion

Now that you've got your lists, look at them side-by-side and start to think about how variations in your causes relate to the symptoms you've listed. Maybe you don't immediately see a relationship. No problem – just spend the next weeks observing how changes in your causes directly affect your symptoms. If you have fibromyalgia, you'll start to see just how closely the causes and symptoms are linked. That is, as your causes improve, you'll also see a parallel improvement in your symptoms. And, of course, should your causes worsen, you can expect your already painful sensations to intensify that much more.

In fact, try a little experiment: take a two-hour break to watch a funny movie. I'll bet your adrenaline level lowers, albeit temporarily, and that you experience some relief from your various aches and pains as a consequence. This will work as long as your fight or flight response will allow you to focus on the movie. I urge you to try many such experiments. It's important that you are observant and give serious thought to the relationships that tie your causes to your symptoms. Learn all that you can, because this information will prove invaluable to you as you work to achieve a cure and reclaim your life. Even this added awareness alone can lead to improvements.

If you haven't already, you should visit your health care provider so you can be tested for certain potentially dangerous causes, including sleep apnea, lupus, and various other painful diseases. Should you have any of these problems, the sooner they can be detected and treated, the better your chances for recovery. Even if the tests for these diseases come back negative, it's still good to rule them out. Also, your doctor may be able to identify certain other medical conditions that play a role in causing your pain and fatigue or interrupting your sleep. For example, perhaps you have a sluggish thyroid gland, which would actually be relatively easy to treat.

Once you're satisfied that you've managed to list all of your causes and each of the symptoms related to your heightened adrenaline level, you are ready to consider the options available to you for treating and curing fibromyalgia:

- **Take medications for comfort.**
- **Utilize treatments that make your body feel better.**
- **Work on your causes to better regulate your adrenaline.**
- **Take medication to better regulate your adrenaline.**

Each of these options were covered extensively in Chapter 5. I'll provide short summaries of each approach here. If you find you still have questions, please feel free to review Chapter 5.

MEDICATIONS FOR COMFORT

Do you need to take something to help you sleep? Most fibromyalgia patients do. Often, this takes the form of over-the-counter sleep aids such as Benadryl or Nytol. Or you can speak with your health care provider to obtain a prescription sleep aid. You may want to ask your doctor whether you should consider medication for depression or anxiety. For some people, pain medications or muscle relaxants may be necessary.

Please remember that while narcotics (such as Vicodin) may provide some temporary relief, the contributions they're able to make to long-term recovery may prove to be marginal at best. Generally speaking, you're likely to realize more long-term benefit from anything you can do to address the causes of your heightened adrenaline level. That said, it's not at all unusual for people to also require some additional symptom relief at first.

In that regard, of all the drug options available to you, I recommend that you place your greatest emphasis on those most likely to help you resume a normal sleep pattern. You may also find that some of the natural remedies and supplements available to you can prove to be quite useful – particularly those associated with treatments for depression, fatigue, sleep-deprivation, and anxiety. Many people find success with natural remedies. Should you choose to explore these options more fully, rest assured that there are many resources available to you. Be sure to discuss your plans with your health care provider. By working together, you should be able to develop a regimen of medications and supplements that will work best for you.

Once you've been able to consult with your health care provider, make a list of all the supplements and medications you plan to take, complete with the daily dose you intend to take and any schedule you might have for increasing that dosage. Use this list to monitor the effectiveness of different drugs and supplements over time.

Prescription Drugs			
Medication	Current Dose	Planned Dose	Beneficial/Adverse Effects

Other Health Supplements			
Medication	Current Dose	Planned Dose	Beneficial/Adverse Effects

TREATMENTS TO MAKE
YOUR BODY FEEL BETTER

Every sensation perceived as amplified by fibromyalgia comes from something that's actually happening in your body. Your central nervous system has simply lost its ability to filter sensations, so you feel them more than you normally would. If the original painful sensation can be reduced, then the amplified signal your brain ultimately experiences is less likely to cause you as much distress. This applies to every sensation, not just aches and pains. This is why some fibromyalgia patients are given injections to reduce pain at key trigger points. Initially, these injections were administered in the mistaken belief that they were the best way to treat "arthritis of the muscles."

We now know that fibromyalgia is no such thing, but since we all are tender wherever our connective tissue comes together, anything that provides relief in those areas can be of value in terms of helping to break the fibromyalgia cycle. This applies not only to trigger point injections, but also to therapeutic massage or any other technique you favor for pain reduction. The cautionary note here, is that on those occasions when you are red-hot with fibromyalgia, you may not be able to tolerate even the lightest of touches.

Whatever your strategy is for reducing pain – be it exercise, massage, bodywork, acupuncture, stretching or even time in a hot tub – always monitor how your body reacts since you may actually be working at cross-purposes to your real objective by creating more sensations to be amplified. The way your body reacts to any sort of stimulation is apt to change on a daily basis. As you continue to monitor your body, you'll become more familiar with the signs of impending trouble and will be much better able to judge when it's time to exercise and when it's time to simply relax.

Review the list below, and place a check mark next to those activities you are currently using to help your body feel better. Circle those activities that you would like to try.

Walking/Exercise

Massage

Acupuncture

Stretching

Ice/Heat

Breathing Exercises

Yoga

Meditation

Craniosacral Therapy

List any additional activities that sound appealing to you but are not listed here:

WORK ON YOUR CAUSES
TO REGULATE YOUR ADRENALINE

Working on your causes is the single best way to treat your fibromyalgia. Go directly after the matter that's at the root of all your other problems – namely, your elevated adrenaline level. Whenever you begin to make changes to lower your adrenaline, your brain will always begin to build back up its dopamine reserves, even if they've been nearly depleted.

I've already asked you to list your causes, so you probably already have a pretty good idea of what's coming next... yes, it's time to start working on those causes. Review your list of causes, and make notes on what types of actions you can take to resolve them. Some causes may be physical in nature and require surgery or other medical treatments. Other causes may be psychological in nature and require a different kind of approach. When it comes to resolving most of your causes, you can probably accomplish a tremendous amount on your own.

Many patients have asked me whether it might be better to just leave well enough alone since they seem to get by as it is. Some go so far as to say that just thinking about fibromyalgia seems to make matters worse. Well, that may be, but if you weren't motivated to get better, I doubt you'd be reading this book. Remember, it's how you think about your fibromyalgia that may affect the problem. If you get stressed thinking about fibromyalgia, it may make it worse.

If, instead, you get excited and start to make a plan to reclaim your life, this will certainly not worsen your fibromyalgia. Also, I know from personal experience that being stuck in a semi-permanent state of high adrenaline is no fun at all. So while it may be true that you're physically able to tolerate the increased adrenaline, you may also be missing out on a great deal of what life has to offer.

Keep in mind that even the most diligent work on your causes is not going to yield a quick fix. That's because this work is a slow and steady process, not an event. And that explains why, in order to obtain quicker relief, there are many who'd like to at least attempt the medications that are part of the off-label protocol discussed in Chapter 5.

It is important to remember that the longer you've suffered with the effects of increased adrenaline, the longer it's going to take your brain to unlearn its reflexive fight or flight way of responding to the outside world.

This is why you may find that improvements come slowly, even if you happen to be making excellent progress in terms of working on your causes. That's when it will be important to remind yourself that even though the improvements may be small, they're long-term improvements because you're in the process of righting your whole limbic system, thus allowing it to operate correctly again for perhaps the first time in many years. This means that over time your sensations will once again be inhibited in a normal manner and that your fatigue and confusion will start to fade away.

At this point in the book, there may be many of you who think that I am just another doctor telling you to be less stressed out and just sleep better. I don't blame you since I promised much more. Although I believe it is easier to work on your causes when provided with an accurate and scientific explanation of how stress causes pain, I have discovered the shortcomings of this approach. Over the years, I have felt a need to go much further into exploring just what's going on inside the human brain; both for my patients and myself. I asked myself a simple question: *Why did we ever get fibromyalgia in the first place?*

The Fight or Flight Response

The fight or flight response is an integral part of our genetic makeup. It's an innate survival instinct that will be with humans until the end of time. Things goes wrong when we use this survival mechanism for psychological threats to our life rather than actual physical threats. As the human species evolved, we found ourselves equipped with basic survival tools. In some species this might be a hard shell, while in others an ability to change colors and blend into the surroundings. Humans were given the greatest protection of all – the most powerful mind of any species – a brain that will look out for us, be our protector and best ally. However, you will only find this to be true if you are able to use your brain appropriately.

How is the brain genetically programmed to operate? Why is your adrenaline up in the first place? What do pain from a motor vehicle accident, interrupted sleep from sleep apnea, and anxiety from post-traumatic stress disorder have in common? A lack of security.

You may not realize this security threat, but certain parts of your brain do. In fact, these parts of your brain may not have felt safe for decades, possibly since you were 3 or 4 years old. The fight or flight response is an innate tool. It can and should be used appropriately. Believe it or not, it is 100 percent in your control to harness the power of your fight or flight response. If you have fibromyalgia, the sad fact is that your fight or flight response is running your life and likely ruining it.

As a previous sufferer of fibromyalgia, I understand the hopelessness you feel. I fully know what a true lack of control feels like. Do you feel hopeless? Is the suffering unbearable with no apparent end in sight? Are you miserable and feel others are enjoying life while you have all the bad luck and have to suffer on the sidelines?

Through my suffering, I found great happiness. In fact, most psychologists know that people won't make drastic changes in their lives until they have enough suffering. This makes sense. Fibromyalgia is true suffering.

I don't have to convince you that your fibromyalgia can be the biggest personal tragedy you have ever had to endure. Through my work, I have found this suffering can be an opportunity for true happiness. You will too.

You only need to make one admission and then you can use your suffering to join me on the road to true happiness. Ask yourself if things are going well or do you want to make drastic changes in the direction your life is going? If you have fibromyalgia, I already know your answer.

Now that you are ready to make some changes, let's learn a little more about the fight or flight response. I believe the fight or flight response is the most important survival instinct we have. Each and every experience we ever have is evaluated by our fight or flight response for any potential security threat. Unfortunately, although our brain is extremely adaptive and capable of tremendous cognitive feats, it was wired for survival in a more primitive world. That doesn't mean we can't survive in a modern world where we're constantly besieged by all manner of stresses and pressures. If the fight or flight response is satisfied, our higher thinking centers will flourish as we think clearly and experience untainted thoughts and emotions. Conversely, if the fight or flight response is not satisfied, we will be quickly directed into our more primitive survival center and will often regress into acting like a threatened animal. This is not necessarily bad and may even be very appropriate. If someone is threatening your children's safety, the fight or flight response will quickly devise a battle plan and help you implement it. However, if someone just cut you off in traffic, it is not very useful to activate your survival center and therefore feel angry and try to attack them – or even simply raise your adrenaline and feel tense and anxious. In the brain, this traffic center may look something like this.

─────── Figure 12 - Higher vs. Primitive Mind ───────

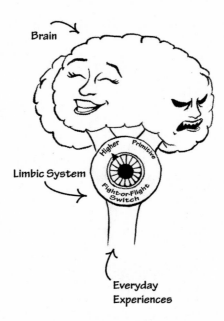

Figure 12 – The limbic system and your fight or flight response have control over how you experience everyday life experiences. And remember, you have control over the fight or flight "switch."

How does your fight or flight response decide which part of your brain will be triggered by a particular experience? Is our response just innate programming? If this were the case, we would all be the same and have exactly the same fears and anxieties. Of course, this isn't the case. So who decides which experience leads to higher thinking centers versus an activation of our primitive survival centers? In other words, where does your brain store the list of what makes you secure and what doesn't? And more importantly, who wrote this list and can it be erased and rewritten?

The list that discerns which experiences provide security and which should threaten you is stored in your limbic system. It is basically the instruction manual for your fight or flight response. Who has control over this list? YOU DO. Your brain wrote this list over your lifetime. It is your instruction manual on how to deal with the world and shapes every experience you ever have.

The subject of my next book and my seminars explains very practical ways of understanding your fight or flight response and using your suffering to begin to rewrite this list. Believe it or not, you can feel secure in the face of lupus or post-traumatic stress disorder. Many will say this takes years of therapy. If this is how long it takes a person to admit that changes need to be made, this may be true. However, if you can use your suffering to take a new radical approach to interpreting the world, you can rewrite your list to find security and great happiness in the face of what used to cause you great suffering.

The purpose of *The Fibromyalgia Cure* is to provide a scientific explanation for fibromyalgia. I believe that once this explanation is accepted, better medications will be developed and better treatments for patients will be possible. If you would like to turn your suffering into personal growth and find true happiness, I invite you to join me at one of my seminars or read my second book. My seminars and next book provide a definitive plan for any person to properly use their fight or flight response.

TAKE MEDICATION TO BETTER REGULATE YOUR ADRENALINE

For those who can tolerate Mirapex and Requip, the odds in your battle against fibromyalgia can suddenly turn dramatically in your favor. The reasons for this are fully explored in Chapter 5. I always encourage my patients to first try to deal with their causes – resorting to dopamine agonists therapy only when it proves to be absolutely necessary. The same logic applies to you.

Even then, you have to approach this protocol knowing full well that there's a good chance you won't be one of the lucky ones able to easily tolerate Mirapex and Requip. Typically, the main problem you will experience is nausea, which, can often be treated and resolved over time. Chances are that new dopamine agonist medications will become available in the near future, which will hopefully be easier for most people to tolerate.

Although Mirapex and Requip are not miracle drugs, they do offer hope to people who are otherwise largely without hope. These are drugs that should only be used as a last resort. If you're looking at taking one of these drugs, you're pretty much already down to your last strike in your battle against fibromyalgia. However, there is a ray of hope, because if you're one of the 50-60 percent who can tolerate the dopamine agonist drugs, you are pretty much assured of getting better. And from a medical standpoint, it's incredibly dramatic to go from being hopeless to having a 50-60 percent shot at recovery on the basis of a single change. That's simply something you don't see all that often in the medical world.

Remember that fibromyalgia does not harm your body in any way, so there's really no need for you to feel rushed into deciding on any one sort of therapy. Certainly, if you have severe fibromyalgia, you'll probably be anxious to attain some relief just as soon as you possibly can. But even then, I wouldn't recommend Mirapex or Requip as your first option.

If your symptoms are mild, I strongly encourage that you put your focus initially on improving your causes. You won't find immediate relief that way, but you can expect slow, steady – and lasting – progress to result. That also means you can keep the dopamine agonists in reserve in the event all else fails. Also, the longer you're able to hold off on taking the dopamine agonists, the better your chances that new, easier-to-tolerate drugs will emerge.

What if nothing works?

If everything you do to mitigate your causes ends up failing and you find you can't tolerate any of the dopamine agonists, don't assume for a moment that the fight is over. Remember, first of all, that fibromyalgia is not causing any permanent harm to your body. The tremendous pain and discomfort you're experiencing is strictly as a consequence of the amplified sensations your central nervous system perceives.

So, first off, you probably need to go back to review your list of causes. Is it possible you've overlooked one? Or did you just fail to see something you didn't want to see? I've had patients, for example, who really needed back surgery, but – for one reason or another – kept putting it off. Well, it turns out that part of the price they ended up paying for that was an intense case of fibromyalgia. In other instances, I've found that a key contributing cause had to do with the fact that a patient was putting off some dreaded decision – for example, whether or not to put an elderly parent into a nursing home. The result there, of course, is that all the mounting stress ends up leaving the person stranded in semi-permanent, fight-or-flight response. This is exactly why I urge anyone who thinks they might be wrestling with psychological causes (including stress) to take the time to learn how to properly use your flight or fight response.

The other ray of hope I can offer is that if you wait long enough, you're may find that your fibromyalgia just ends up getting better on its own. That's because, as your circumstances change, it's possible the sources of stress contributing to your fibromyalgia will also change, or maybe even disappear altogether. Perhaps life will become more secure or your rheumatoid arthritis will go into remission.

Once fibromyalgia goes away, can it come back?

Once you find that you're getting better and your causes improve, you may find that you're able to safely lower your dose of Mirapex or Requip. That's especially true, if your case of fibromyalgia is one that was triggered by events that are already behind you (a divorce that happened several years ago, for example) and your use of Mirapex or Requip was really just intended to help break your vicious cycle. In general, you can start weaning yourself off the drugs a few months after you're quite certain your causes are gone.

Just be aware that anything that serves to drive your adrenaline level back up again may cause a flare-up. Should that happen, review the four approaches laid out in this book for treating fibromyalgia – and then, put your emphasis on whatever it is that worked best for you the first time around.

After recovery, some of my patients have actually become depressed once they got better. That's because they started to mourn the time they lost and all the opportunities they missed while they were struggling with fibromyalgia. For some, there are even lost marriages and friendships to grieve over. This mourning is perfectly understandable, but as you start to become consumed in your grief, your adrenaline level is virtually guaranteed to start rising again. And so, the more you grieve what you've lost in the past, the greater the chance that you'll have even more things to mourn in the future.

Instead, why not celebrate your liberation from an affliction that's trapped and tormented you for months or years. You've managed to get your life back! What's more, you've succeeded in overcoming your primitive fight or flight response. That makes you a more highly evolved person, one who's now better able to properly use your fight or flight response.

Put another way, you are now able to manage your fight or flight response, whereas before it was the other way around. And for making this life-affirming breakthrough, I congratulate you.

The key lesson is that it is never too late to get your life back.

For those of us who've managed to recover fully, the lingering gift is that – once you've lived through all the suffering that fibromyalgia brings – you're much better able to appreciate all the wonderful things life has to offer.

CONCLUSION

No one is immune to fibromyalgia. All it takes is a sufficient accumulation of causes to make someone a hostage of their own adrenaline system. That said, fibromyalgia should not be thought of as a disease. It's a matter of heightened sensations that owes to a diminished supply of dopamine in the brain.

The problem is that the brain can't tell the difference between a physical threat to your life and a psychological threat. Both will result in elevated adrenaline levels. Besides leading to more suffering, this can also be the source of tremendous unhappiness. That's because when people are running on high adrenaline, the basic survival centers of the brain take control, effectively locking you into the fight or flight response. For some, this can lead directly to anger and violence. For others, fibromyalgia is the result. It's even thought that cancer and many infections may stem, at least in part, from chronically elevated adrenaline levels.

It's my hope that the medical community will come to better understand and appreciate the mind-body link. Adrenaline certainly plays a key role here, but it's probably not alone. There are also other brain chemicals that may play a role in physical diseases such as heart attacks and cancer. With better understanding of the mind-body link, we should eventually find the brain chemicals responsible for the placebo effect often seen in clinical trials.

I am pleased with the dopamine research that's been done in recent years on the basis of stress tests in lab rats. Similar tests should be run with humans, using PET scans and other monitoring techniques. In all likelihood, this would allow us to develop better, more specific therapies than Mirapex and Requip offer today. I also think these tests would shed light on some other related conditions such as irritable bowel syndrome.

Fibromyalgia, like any other medical condition, can and should be thoroughly understood through science. Only through science can fibromyalgia ever gain recognition as a legitimate and widespread medical condition that affects tens of millions of people around the world. Beyond the scientific explanation of fibromyalgia, it's imperative for people to understand that you cannot solve the problems of the body without solving the problems of the mind. It's been a personal life goal of mine to give scientific legitimacy to the mind-body connection. I hope that this book stimulates intense curiosity for anyone wanting to understand this connection. My next book, *Taking Control of Your Fight or Flight Response: An Instruction Manual for the Human Brain*, will satisfy the questions raised in *The Fibromyalgia Cure*. Through science, this book unlocks the genetic programming of human behavior and uses the lessons learned to show anyone how to properly use their fight or flight response.

Appendix for Healthcare Providers

When I told my colleagues that I was writing this book, they frequently asked the following question: "These patients are the biggest drain on my time, and it is nearly always a disappointing experience for both patient and provider. Why would I ever choose to treat a fibromyalgia patient?"

In the past I would have been the first to agree with them. I spent fourteen years being trained to think like this. The medical community has honestly tried to help fibromyalgia patients, but until now we had no answers to the questions that any physician wants to know when treating a patient: What is it? What will it do to the patient? How can I treat it?

Now that I understand the science of fibromyalgia, I can provide you with a plan for any patient with fibromyalgia. For those patients that fail symptomatic treatment and are unable to work on the causes of this syndrome, I prescribe the dopamine agonists Mirapix and/or Requip. I prescribe these drugs following the off-label protocol originally developed by Dr. Andrew Holman and confirmed in my own clinic. These drugs are virtually 100 percent effective for these patients, but difficult to tolerate. This is fully explained at the end of this appendix. With time, you can become an expert in understanding the fibromyalgia syndrome and in prescribing the dopamine agonists.

The most satisfying thing for me is to have a solid understanding of the syndrome. Every patient I see can be fully understood and given a definitive plan to follow. Over time, it becomes clearer what symptoms fibromyalgia is causing and what it is not.

Fibromyalgia is not a somatization disorder. Many of my patients have had neuropsychological evaluations and the diagnosis is usually somatization disorder. *Up to Date* describes somatization disorder as follows:

> Somatization refers to the tendency to experience psychological distress in the form of somatic symptoms and to seek medical help for these symptoms. Emotional responses such as anxiety and depression initiate and/or perpetuate symptoms. A diagnosed physical illness does not account for the symptoms, nor do the symptoms seem in proportion to what would be seen in a diagnosed illness.
>
> Somatization can be conscious or unconscious and may be influenced by psychological distress or a desire for personal gain. Somatization contributes to more frequent use of medical services and to frustration in both the patient and the doctor.[1]

This is more likely describing fibromyalgia. I doubt there ever was such a thing as somatization disorder. When a patient is diagnosed with somatization disorder, they are told nothing is really happening, and that they are somehow imagining the symptoms. Of course the symptoms do not seem "in proportion to what would be seen in a diagnosed illness." In fibromyalgia, the sensations that the patient is noticing are actually occurring. However, they are perceived as amplified in the central nervous system. We now have scientific proof of just how the causes of fibromyalgia affect the brain and deplete dopamine. Once this knowledge becomes more mainstream, it is my hope that somatization disorder will become a thing of the past.

After reading this book and better understanding how fibromyalgia works, you will more easily be able to diagnose fibromyalgia patients. These patients will have confidence in you when you can fully explain their fibromyalgia. You will be able to list their particular causes, explain which symptoms are from the fibromyalgia and which are not, and give them a definitive plan for relief. You will even look forward to these patients coming in for their appointment, as they can become the most gratifying patients you have ever treated. I look forward to my fibromyalgia patients as "catch up" patients in the midst of a day filled with complicated rheumatological patients.

To make things simpler, the diagnostic criteria can be condensed into four categories:

- **Sleep**
- **Psychological**
- **Pain**
- **Related (RLS, hypermobility)**

In order to be diagnosed with fibromyalgia, patients must have the causes described in Chapter 2 and their fatigue, confusion, and amplified sensations must vary with these causes. If they have other problems that cause pain, such as tendonitis or arthritis, these are likely amplified by their fibromyalgia.

In general, if you can't easily identify obvious causes, the patient either doesn't have fibromyalgia, or they have hidden medical causes such as lupus or sleep apnea. Keep in mind that if a patient has lupus or rheumatoid arthritis, they are already half the way to developing fibromyalgia. Poor sleep, depression, or stress will add to increased adrenaline levels, and fibromyalgia may soon develop.

If one tender point hurts much more than the others, it could be tendonitis or bursitis on top of fibromyalgia. Fibromyalgia patients will notice even the slightest inflammation when the sensations are perceived as amplified. This may even bring a cancer to attention earlier, but usually leads to much negative testing instead.

There are four potential ways to treat fibromyalgia:

1) Prescribe medications for immediate relief.
2) Recommend treatments that make the body feel better.
3) Work on the causes in order to restore dopamine levels.
4) Prescribe medications to restore dopamine levels.

Medications for immediate relief.

The most important thing you can ever do for a patient with fibromyalgia is to explain to them what they have, what causes it, and what can be done. The most important thing you can prescribe for them is a dopamine agonist. However, of all the standard medications, something for sleep is the most important. In order to normalize the adrenaline cycle, trazodone or benzodiazepines can be a real help. I prescribe trazodone first, but quickly follow with Xanax or Ativan if the trazodone is not effective. In order to be effective, these medications may require take higher doses than normal in a fibromyalgia patient. I avoid Elavil due to the associated weight gain and dry mouth. Of course, patients can become dependent on any sleep medication. However, if the patient is unable to work on their causes and wants medication, I find something for sleep is the best place to start.

Pain medications are useful, but as described in Chapter 5, they may not be effective. I usually prescribe 3-4 Vicodin a day and stop there. The best pain medication is generally Mirapex. There are many other medications for comfort. Some physicians prescribe anti-depressants for fibromyalgia patients. However, if the patient is not depressed, anti-depressants will do little for their fibromyalgia.

Treatments that make the body feel better.

Fibromyalgia results in fatigue, confusion, and amplified sensations. The more underlying problems are calmed down in the body, the less they will hurt when the resulting sensations are perceived as amplified. The patient should first work on their causes and then try a dopamine agonist, but if neither of these is successful the patient may need trigger point injections or surgery. Every underlying problem will be amplified, so if you can't fix the amplification, the problem will have to be treated.

In fibromyalgia, surgery can be very helpful if used to treat an underlying medical condition. However, many patients don't get better like they should. As previously pointed out, even the slightest hint of a residual problem after surgery will be amplified. This must be taken into account before the patient is brought into the operating room. I am in no way discouraging operating on a patient with fibromyalgia. I would just rather try to fix the low levels of dopamine in the brain first, and then see what we are left with. Although I rarely use local trigger point injections, these can also be quite helpful at times.

In addition, anything that makes the body feel better should be encouraged. This was outlined in Chapter 5, and includes chiropractic, physical therapy, heat, and many other modalities. Remember, if they are red hot with fibromyalgia, they might not tolerate any exercise or even light touch, but if the symptoms are calmed down, even deep massage can be very helpful. It will be up to the patient to determine what they can tolerate. You can also judge this by counting and rating their tender points. These are graded on the following scale:

½ - mild pain (most people can have this)

1 - pain

2 - winces in pain

3 - withdraws from your four pounds of pressure-
    this means just until the blood begins to leave
    your fingernail.

The amount of residual pain in a trigger point can be used to judge your treatment's effectiveness.

Work on or treat causes in order to regulate their adrenaline.
Identifying and treating the causes of fibromyalgia is the best thing the best thing you can do for your patients. Help them identify the causes and develop a plan to begin resolving them. This can range from dealing with stress, prescribing medications for anxiety or panic disorders, or recommending the back surgery they were putting off. Whatever is increasing their adrenaline from my list of causes should be resolved as much as possible. The single best way to treat fibromyalgia is to teach patients how to properly use their fight or flight response. More information is available on this topic at www.drdryland.com.

If patients have trouble with sleep, I ask them to purchase *Say Goodnight to Insomnia*. I also ask every patient about sleep apnea. An overnight oximetry study is cheap and can catch many cases of sleep apnea. However, if the suspicion of sleep apnea is high, especially in men, the patient should be sent for a formal sleep study. Even subtle cases of sleep apnea can add to the vicious cycle of fibromyalgia.

Most patients need to be examined for degenerative and inflammatory arthritis, as these are common causes of fibromyalgia. Anything that causes pain can raise adrenaline levels and cause secondary fibromyalgia. I have seen cases of fibromyalgia resolve with Methotrexate alone in patients that have lupus. This adds to the complexity of fibromyalgia, and it takes experience to distinguish fibromyalgia from other pains.

Pain syndromes are ever changing, and whenever things aren't going that well I have to ask myself the question "What pain am I currently treating?" At any point it can be the inflammatory arthritis or the fibromyalgia. This is actually somewhat easy to figure out if we go back to the causes of fibromyalgia. If the patient's causes got worse and their exam is suggestive of worsening tender points, then it is probably a fibromyalgia flare. On the other hand, if their causes haven't changed, then it may be that the inflammatory arthritis is under-treated. I would say that I see secondary fibromyalgia in about 75 percent of my lupus patients and 33 percent of patients with rheumatoid arthritis. It is present in over 90 percent of elderly patients with severe generalized osteoarthritis.

Many doctors ask me how to know what pains are from the arthritis and what pains are from the fibromyalgia. With time and better treatment, it becomes easier to tell these apart. In addition, the patient can keep track and determine which pains vary with their fibromyalgia causes and which do not. Many patients will say that the fibromyalgia feels like it is in the muscles and the other feels like it is in the joints, but this can be misleading in many cases.

In general, if prednisone or NSAIDs are very helpful, then you are probably treating something else besides the fibromyalgia. I often do a 2-3 week trial of prednisone in patients with a positive ANA and fibromyalgia while I am waiting for the results of the labs and x-rays I ordered at their initial visit. In addition, if there is severe fatigue or confusion associated with the pain, fibromyalgia is much more likely.

Once the diagnosis of fibromyalgia is sound, I treat their medical condition as outlined above. However, many patients have both fibromyalgia and something else causing pain. In these cases, I begin by treating the causes, such as lupus and/or interrupted sleep. If the patient still has significant fibromyalgia when the underlying causes are treated, then I also maximally treat their fibromyalgia.

As any sensation can be amplified in fibromyalgia, the patient will notice problems in the body earlier. These problems will be more bothersome, harder to treat and last longer. This can range from annoying edema, which most people wouldn't notice, all the way to an early nodule that turns out to be lymphoma.

Unfortunately, this leads to more testing and it can be a real struggle to know when to stop worrying that you are missing something. This is why I always go back to the same game plan. Treat the fibromyalgia. The patient will then stop perceiving amplified sensations and we can see what other medical conditions we are left with.

If the patient has overwhelming psychological causes of fibromyalgia, you may need to refer them to a psychiatrist or therapist. I have found that patients are much more willing to do this once they realize that if they deal with the psychological causes, this will directly reduce the amount of fatigue, confusion, and amplified sensations that they currently experience. This may take years of therapy, but every small improvement will lower their adrenaline and begin to break the vicious cycle of fibromyalgia they have been stuck in for years. Even just explaining to them what fibromyalgia truly is can lower their anxiety over what is happening to them and begin to lower their adrenaline. I find that at least 20 percent of patients don't even want treatment once they understand fibromyalgia and the fact that it is not causing permanent physiological damage in any way.

Many doctors have expressed frustration in the unwillingness of some patients to find professional psychiatric help. I encourage patients to take this approach by explaining that they simply need to do whatever they can to lower their adrenaline. This may mean getting back surgery, working only the day shift, or seeing a psychiatrist. They simply need to work on their causes. This is always the best way to treat fibromyalgia.

Prescribe medications to regulate their adrenaline.
One of the most satisfying experience I have ever had as a physician was the first time I prescribed Mirapix to a fibromyalgia patient. She came back two months later and told me that she got her life back. She couldn't stop thanking me and I was only more encouraged to learn everything I could about the dopamine ago-

nists. Anyone can become a local expert in treating fibromyalgia by studying this book and gaining experience in the use of dopamine agonists. Please design your own consent form and once comfortable, try to prescribe it yourself.

If you want to pick the best candidate, find a young patient with few GI complaints and you will likely have at least 90 percent tolerance. The drugs are poorly tolerated when they are prescribed to everyone without considering age, GI sx's, and h/o multiple medication intolerances. If you choose your patients wisely and give ginger, phenergan or strong acid blockers, the tolerance can approach 90 percent. However, I try dopamine agonists in virtually all patients. Sometimes I am surprised at who tolerates them and I am glad I tried.

Find your own comfort level and I will try to answer provider's questions about the use of these medications on my website: www.drdryland.com. These medications, along with all of the ways to treat fibromyalgia discussed in this book should save the healthcare system a tremendous amount of money. This is what I have found to be the case in most of my patients, especially the ones that tolerate dopamine agonists or successfully treat their causes.

Even with everything I have learned about fibromyalgia, I am still stuck in about 20 percent of cases. These are patients who have severe fibromyalgia and are unable to work on their causes. They find little relief in medications for comfort and are unable to make things in their body feel better as they can't even tolerate light touch. They are also unable to tolerate the dopamine agonists and have a long history of medication intolerances. They are stuck in the vicious cycle of fibromyalgia, depression, anxiety and poor sleep, which only leads to an intensification of their fibromyalgia.

In these patients, I explain again that they are not being harmed in any way and fibromyalgia is just fatigue, confusion, and amplified sensations. Just reminding them about this can lead to a lessening of their anxiety. Then I simply go back to the only four ways to treat fibromyalgia.

1) Prescribe medications for immediate relief.
2) Recommend treatments that make the body feel better.
3) Work on the causes in order to restore dopamine levels.
4) Prescribe medications to restore dopamine levels.

I have a few hundred patients that are waiting for the next specific dopamine agonist to be released. There are some in the pipeline. Hopefully with my book, along with Dr. Andrew Holman's upcoming book, and current lab research being done on stress and the brain, the pharmaceutical companies will take a closer look at this class of drugs. There are currently more patients with fibromyalgia than rheumatoid arthritis and lupus combined and the number continues to grow.

Short of the next new dopamine agonist, patients still have to work on their causes. Once the medications are maximized and they are doing things for comfort, then the patient must take a hard look at their causes if they want relief. This may mean going back to get a better mask for their CPAP machine or making drastic changes in their life to avoid stress and whatever else is raising their adrenaline.

The best overall thing any patient can do is to learn how to properly use their fight or flight response. To date, there are not very many resources in the medical community for my patients on treating an overactive fight or flight response. As I began to question what truly raises patient's sympathetic tone, I realized that the fight of flight response was not properly understood. My research on this topic is fully explained in my upcoming book *Taking Control of Your Fight or Flight Response: An Instruction Manual for the Human Brain.*

Off-label protocol for dopamine agonists.

When prescribing Mirapix, I usually start patients with a mild test dose to be administered for the first 2-3 weeks while I wait for any other test results to return from the lab. Typically, this means an initial dose of just 0.125 mg a day, taken just before bedtime. I'll then step up the daily dosage by 0.125 mg with each passing week while I monitor how the patient responds as we progress up to 0.375 mg per night. Assuming the response to the medication is good (they can tolerate it), I'll then launch into the full protocol – with 0.5 mg tabs being prescribed for nightly usage. Thereafter, I step up the daily dosage by a half tab, which is .25 mg, with each passing week. After eight more weeks, patients who are doing well with the drug should be increased up to 2 mg per night. At this point, I switch them to 1.5 mg tabs and continue to methodically increase the dosage in 0.75 mg increments every two weeks. The goal is to get each patient up to 4.5 mg a night.

If necessary, this stepwise increase in dosage can be slowed. Also, for those who manage to make headway against their fibromyalgia at lower doses, there's really no reason to step up the dosage. You can always do that later should progress slow or plateau at any point. Also, should it turn out that the maximum dose of Mirapex tolerated isn't quite enough to rein in your patient's symptoms, you should consider supplementing it with Requip.

Generally, in such instances, I start out patients with 1 mg daily doses of Requip and then step up the protocol by 1 mg a week. By and large, the Requip dose needs to be three times larger than the Mirapex dose to net the same effect. For example, if your patient can only tolerate 1.5 mg of Mirapex a day – instead of the optimal 4.5 mg – then you should probably aim to replace the missing 3 mg with 9 mg of Requip. It will take the patient at least 9 weeks to reach that level.

Requip can also be used on its own, in which case I'd recommend starting with .25 mg, then ramping up to .75 mg. If this is tolerated, the patient should then take 1 mg each night, increasing to a nightly maximum of 12-15 mg over a like number of weeks. In general, patients who find they can't tolerate Mirapex at all still have a reasonable chance of being able to handle Requip.

There's no disputing that nausea as a side-effect is unpleasant, but it can generally be treated effectively with ginger or medications such as Phenergan, Compazine, and Zofran. In addition, acid blockers such as Prilosec, Pepto Bismol, or Pepcid-ac can be quite helpful. For even more assistance, you may want to consider prescribing Nexium (up to 40 mg three times a day) or Prevacid (30 mg up to three times a day). It's also very important to maintain a consistent regimen, since some patients can experience extreme nausea should they take a break before restarting the medications. If the patient ends up skipping a few days, they may need to rebuild the dosage slowly again, albeit not quite as slowly as the first time.

In my view, "tolerating the medication," means few or no side effects. And that's important — not simply because of comfort, but also because interrupted sleep and severe nausea are unlikely to help the adrenaline cycle improve. Patients should definitely stop the medications if they experience any major side effects or find that the side effects aren't resolving promptly.

Another point worth noting is that these medications should not be stopped abruptly in the event they are being taken at high doses. It is possible that a rare side effect similar to Neuroleptic Malignant Syndrome, which can bring on fever, confusion, low blood pressure and shortness of breath, could occur. Patients should always be weaned off these medications over a few days to a week. Although there are no recorded instances of Neuroleptic Malignant Syndrome associated with Mirapex or Requip usage, it has been noted with other drugs of the same pharmacological family.

There are those who take a dim view of using drugs to manipulate brain chemistry. I understand this perspective, but unfortunately that would leave some fibromyalgia sufferers without any options. Also, I find it hard to accept that replacing a depleted supply of dopamine is in some way tantamount to "tampering with nature." I wonder how natural it is for a person to be faced with living their whole life stuck in their fight or flight response. For me, the choice is easy. I'll never tell a fibromyalgia patient who's unable to work and whose life is disintegrating that it's wrong to regulate their adrenaline levels through the use of medications. My instinct, and my humanity, dictates instead that I congratulate the patient for being courageous enough to do whatever it takes to reclaim their life.

The following pages include a sample consent form for prescribing Mirapex and/or Requip when treating fibromyalgia.

Informed Consent
for the
Administration of Medication

On _____ I had a conversation with

Dr. _____ and he/she discussed the issues of this document:

I understand that my doctor, in diagnosing my condition, has included fibromyalgia.

As part of my treatment, Dr. _____ has recommended I be given the following

Medication(s): Mirapex and/or Requip

1. Treatment Alternatives: The treatment alternatives include: analgesics, non-steroidal anti-inflammatory agents, sleeping medications, muscle relaxants, and/or anti-depressants.

2. Risks: This authorization is given with the understanding that any treatment involves some risks and hazards. I understand that it is not possible to anticipate all side effects.

Some significant and substantial risks of this particular treatment were discussed earlier with emphasis on sleepiness, anxiety, tremor, worsening sleep, vivid dreams, confusion, hallucinations, light-headedness, hair loss, agitation, fluid retention, and tremulousness. I was also informed that the use of Mirapex and/or Requip for fibromyalgia is not approved by the Food and Drug Administration. It's use for the treatment of fibromyalgia is considered experimental and off-label. I also have had it explained that some possible unknown side effects could happen when the drug is used at high doses for conditions other than Parkinson's disease.

3. Special Instructions: As a result of some of the potential side effects, you are advised not to operate a motor vehicle or heavy machinery if sleepy or confused. Even if not sleepy or confused, you should still make a special effort to drive a vehicle only with extreme caution.

4. Pregnancy should be avoided while receiving the above medication.

5. Tagamet (cimetidine) should not be used in conjunction with Mirapex.

146

6. Ciprofloxacin should not be used in conjunction with Requip. Other medications can interact with Requip and I will always discuss all medications used with Dr. _____.

IF YOU HAVE ANY QUESTIONS AS TO THE RISKS OR HAZARDS OF THE PROPOSED TREATMENT, OR ANY QUESTIONS CONCERNED THE PROPOSED TREATMENT, ASK YOUR PHYSICIAN NOW BEFORE SIGNING THIS CONSENT FORM!

DO NOT SIGN UNLESS YOU HAVE READ AND THOROUGHLY UNDERSTAND THIS FORM!

PATIENT'S CONSENT: I have read and fully understand this consent form. I understand I should not sign this form if treatment alternatives, risks and special instructions have not been explained to my satisfaction. I further understand that I should not sign this form if I have unanswered questions or if I do not understand any of the terms or words used in this consent form. I give my consent to the administration of the above named medications.

If I decide to stop taking the medications, I will contact my physician right away.

_____   _____

Patient/ Responsible Party   Date

_____   _____

Witness   Date

7. PHYSICIAN DECLARATION: I have explained the contents of this document to the patient and have answered all the patient's questions, and to the best of my knowledge, I feel the patient has been adequately informed and has consented.

_____   _____

Physician's Signature   Date

NOTES

Chapter 2

1. Simms, R., S. Roy, M. Hrovat, et al., "Lack of association between fibromyalgia syndrome and abnormalities in muscle energy metabolism." Arthritis & Rheumatism 37 (1994): 794-800.

2. Martinez-Lavin, M., A. Hermosillo, M. Rosas, M. Soto, "Circadian studies of autonomic nervous balance in patients with fibromyalgia" *Arthritis & Rheumatism* 41 (1998): 1966-1971.

   Cohen, H., L. Neumann, A. Alhosshle, et al., "Abnormal sympathovagal balance in men with fibromyalgia." *Journal of Rheumatology* 28 (2001): 581-589.

   Mountz, J, L. Bradley, G. Alarco, "Abnormal functional activity of the central nervous system in fibromyalgia syndrome." *American Journal of Medical Sciences* 315 (1998): 385-396.

   Vaeroy, H., Z. Qiao, L. Morkrid, et al., "Altered sympathetic nervous system response in patients with fibromyalgia." *Journal of Rheumatology* 16 (1989): 1460-1465.

3. Raj, S., D. Brouillard, C. Simpson, et al., "Dysautonomia among patients with fibromyalgia: a noninvasive assessment." *Journal of Rheumatology* 27 (2000): 2660-2665.

4. Routtinen, H., M. Partinen, C. Hublin, et al., "An FDOPA PET study in patients with periodic limb movement disorder and restless legs syndrome." *Neurology* 54 (2000): 502-504.

   Turjanski, N., A. Lees, D. Brooks, "Striatal dopaminergic function in restless legs syndrome." *Neurology* 52 (1999): 932-937.

5. Yunus, M., J. Aldag, "Restless legs syndrome and leg cramps in fibromyalgia syndrome: a controlled study." *British Medical Journal* 312 (1996): 1339.

6. Holman, A., "Safety and efficacy of the dopamine agonist, pramipexole, on pain score for refractory fibromyalgia." *Arthritis & Rheumatism* (Supplement) 43 (2000): S333.

7. Altier, N., J. Stewart, "The role of dopamine in the nucleus accumbens in analgesia." *Life Sciences* 65 (1999): 2269-2287.

8. Torres, I., S. Cucco, M. Bassani, et al. "Long-lasting hyperalgesia after chronic restraint stress in rats-effect of morphine administration." *Neuroscience Research* 45 (2003): 277-283.

9. Gambarana, C. F. Mas, A. Tagliamonte, et al., "A chronic stress that impairs reactivity in rats also decreases dopaminergic transmission in the nucleus accumbens: a microdialysis study." *Journal of Neurochemistry* 72 (1999): 2039-2046.

Quintero, L., M. Moreno, C. Avila, et al., "Long-lasting delayed hyperalgesia after subchronic swim stress." *Pharmacology Biochemistry and Behavior* 67 (2000): 449-458.

Snow, A., S. Tucker, W. Dewey, "The role of neurotransmitters in stress-induced antinociception" *Pharmacolcogy, Biochemistry & Behavior* 16 (1982): 47-50.

Chapter 3

1. Moldofsky, H., P. Scarisbrick, "Induction of neurasthenic musculoskeletal pain syndrome by selective sleep stage deprivation." *Psychosomatic Medicine* 38 (1976): 35-44.

2. Affleck, G., S. Urrows, H. Tennen, et al., "Sequential daily relations of sleep, pain intensity, and attention to pain among women with fibromyalgia." *Pain* 68 (1996): 363-368.

3. May, K., S. West, M. Baker, et al., "Sleep apnea in male patients with the fibromyalgia syndrome." *The American Journal of Medicine* 94 (1993): 505-508.

4. Pellegrino, M., "Atypical chest pain as an initial presentation of primary fibromyalgia." *Archives of Physical Medicine & Rehabilitation* 71 (1990): 526-528.

Chapter 4

1. Davis, J., L. Loh, J. Nodal, et al., "Effects of sleep on the pattern of CO_2 stimulated breathing in males and females." Proceedings of the Symposium on Regulation of Respiration During Sleep and Anesthesia held at the Faculté de Médecine Saint-Antoine, Paris, France, July 14-16, 1977.

2. Taylor, S., L. Klein, B. Lewis, et al., "Biobehavioral responses to stress in females: tend-and-befriend, not fight-or-flight." *Psychological Review* 107 (2000): 411-429.

3. Dick, B., C. Eccleston, G. Crombez, "Attentional functioning in fibromyalgia, rheumatoid arthritis, and musculoskeletal pain patients." *Arthritis and Rheumatism: Arthritis Care and Research* 47 (2002): 639-644.

   Glass, J., D. Park, "Cognitive dysfunction in fibromyalgia." *Current Rheumatology Reports* 3 (2001):123-127.

   Landro, N., T. Stiles, H. Sletvold, "Memory functioning in patients with primary fibromyalgia and major depression and healthy controls." *Journal of Psychosomatic Research* 42 (1997): 297-306.

4. Newcomer, J., G. Selke, A. Melson, et al., "Decreased memory performance in healthy humans induced by stress-level Cortisol treatment." *Archives of General Psychiatry* 56 (1999): 527-533.

Chapter 5

1. Torres, I., S. Cucco, M. Bassani, et al., "Long-lasting hyperalgesia after chronic restraint stress in rats-effect of morphine administration." *Neuroscience Research* 45 (2003): 277-283.

2. Holman, A., "Safety and efficacy of the dopamine agonist, pramipexole, on pain score for refractory fibromyalgia." *Arthritis & Rheumatism* (Supplement) 43 (2000): S333.

Chapter 7

1. Moldofsky, H., P. Scarisbrick, "Induction of neurasthenic musculoskeletal pain syndrome by selective sleep stage deprivation." *Psychosomatic Medicine* 38 (1976): 35-44.

Wood, P., "Stress and dopamine: implications for the pathophysiology of chronic widespread pain." *Medical Hypotheses* 62 (2004): 420-424.

BIBLIOGRAPHY

Affleck, G., S. Urrows, H. Tennen, P. Higgins, Abeles. "Sequential daily relations of sleep, pain intensity, and attention to pain among women with fibromyalgia." *Pain* 68 (1996): 363-368.

Altier, N., J. Stewart, "The role of dopamine in the nucleus accumbens in analgesia." *Life Sciences* 65 (1999): 2269-2287.

Altier, N., J. Stewart, "The Tachykinin NK-1 receptor antagonist, RP-67580, infused into the ventral tegmental area prevents stress-induced analgesia in the formalin test." *Physiology & Behavior* 66 (1999): 717-721.

Cohen, H., L. Neumann, A. Alhosshle, M. Kotler, M. Abu-Shakra, D. Buskila, "Abnormal sympathovagal balance in men with fibromyalgia." *Journal of Rheumatology* 28 (2001): 581-589.

Davis, J., L. Loh, J. Nodal, et al., "Effects of sleep on the pattern of CO_2 stimulated breathing in males and females." Proceedings of the Symposium on Regulation of Respiration During Sleep and Anesthesia held at the Faculté de Médecine Saint-Antoine, Paris, France, July 14-16, 1977.

Dick, B., C. Eccleston, G. Crombez, "Attentional functioning in fibromyalgia, rheumatoid arthritis, and musculoskeletal pain patients." *Arthritis and Rheumatism: Arthritis Care and Research* 47 (2002): 639-644.

Gambarana, C. F. Mas, A. Tagliamonte, A. Scheggi, O. Ghiglieri, M. De Montis, "A chronic stress that impairs reactivity in rats also decreases dopaminergic transmission in the nucleus accumbens: a microdialysis study." *Journal of Neurochemistry* 72 (1999): 2039-2046.

Glass, J., D. Park, "Cognitive dysfunction in fibromyalgia." *Current Rheumatology Reports* 3 (2001):123-127.

Holman, A., "Safety and efficacy of the dopamine agonist, pramipexole, on pain score for refractory fibromyalgia." *Arthritis & Rheumatism* (Supplement) 43 (2000): S333.

Kalivas, P., P. Duffy, "Selective activation of dopamine transmission in the shell of the nucleus accumbens by stress." *Brain Research* 675 (1995): 325-328.

Landro, N., T. Stiles, H. Sletvold, "Memory functioning in patients with primary fibromyalgia and major depression and healthy controls." *Journal of Psychosomatic Research* 42 (1997): 297-306.

Martinez-Lavin, M., A. Hermosillo, M. Rosas, M. Soto, "Circadian studies of autonomic nervous balance in patients with fibromyalgia" *Arthritis & Rheumatism* 41 (1998): 1966-1971.

May, K., S. West, M. Baker, D. Everett, "Sleep apnea in male patients with the fibromyalgia syndrome." *The American Journal of Medicine* 94 (1993): 505-508.

Moldofsky, H., P. Scarisbrick, "Induction of neurasthenic musculoskeletal pain syndrome by selective sleep stage deprivation." *Psychosomatic Medicine* 38 (1976): 35-44.

Mountz, J, L. Bradley, G. Alarcon, "Abnormal functional activity of the central nervous system in fibromyalgia syndrome." *American Journal of Medical Sciences* 315 (1998): 385-396.

Newcomer, J., G. Selke, A. Melson, T. Hershey, S. Craft, K. Richards, A. Alderson, "Decreased memory performance in healthy humans induced by stress-level Cortisol treatment." *Archives of General Psychiatry* 56 (1999): 527-533.

Pellegrino, M., "Atypical chest pain as an initial presentation of primary fibromyalgia." *Archives of Physical Medicine & Rehabilitation* 71 (1990): 526-528.

Quintero, L., M. Moreno, C. Avila, J. Arcaya, W. Maixner, H. Suarez-Roca, "Long-lasting delayed hyperalgesia after subchronic swim stress." *Pharmacology, Biochemistry and Behavior* 67 (2000): 449-458.

Raj, S., D. Brouillard, C. Simpson, W. Hopman, H. Abdollah, "Dysautonomia among patients with fibromyalgia: a noninvasive assessment." *Journal of Rheumatology* 27 (2000): 2660-2665.

Routtinen, H., M. Partinen, C. Hublin, J. Bergman, M. Haaparanta, O. Solin, J. Rinne, "An FDOPA PET study in patients with periodic limb movement disorder and restless legs syndrome." *Neurology* 54 (2000): 502-504.

Schegg, S., B. Leggio, F. Masi, S. Grappi, C. Gambarana, G. Nann, R. Rauggi, M. DeMontis, "Selective modifications in the nucleus accumbens of dopamine synaptic transmission in rats exposed to chronic stress." *Journal of Neurochemistry* 83(2002): 895-903.

Simms, R., S. Roy, M. Hrovat, J. Anderson, G. Skrinar, S. LePoole, C. Zerbini, C. DeLuca, F. Jolesz, "Lack of association between fibromyalgia syndrome and abnormalities in muscle energy metabolism." *Arthritis & Rheumatism* 37 (1994): 794-800.

Snow, A., S. Tucker, W. Dewey, "The role of neurotransmitters in stress-induced antinociception" *Pharmacolcogy, Biochemistry & Behavior* 16 (1982): 47-50.

Taylor, S., L. Klein, B. Lewis, T. Gruenewald, R.Gurung, J. Updegraff, "Biobehavioral responses to stress in females: tend-and-befriend, not fight-or-flight." *Psychological Review* 107 (2000): 411-429.

Torres, I., S. Cucco, M. Bassani, M. Duarte, P. Silveira, A. Vasconcellos, A. Tabajara, G. Dantas, F. Fontella, C. Dalmaz, M. Ferreira, "Long-lasting hyperalgesia after chronic restraint stress in rats-effect of morphine administration." *Neuroscience Research* 45 (2003): 277-283.

Turjanski, N., A. Lees, D. Brooks, "Striatal dopaminergic function in restless legs syndrome." *Neurology* 52 (1999): 932-937.

Wood, P., "Stress and dopamine: implications for the pathophysiology of chronic widespread pain." *Medical Hypotheses* 62 (2004): 420-424.

Vaeroy, H., Z. Qiao, L. Morkrid, O. Forre, "Altered sympathetic nervous system response in patients with fibromyalgia." *Journal of Rheumatology* 16 (1989): 1460-1465.

Yunus, M., J. Aldag, "Restless legs syndrome and leg cramps in fibromyalgia syndrome: a controlled study." *British Medical Journal* 312 (1996): 1339.

Printed in the United States
27321LVS00003BA/88-408

9 780976 649007